STRONG
IN THE
BROKEN
PLACES

PRAISE FOR *STRONG IN THE BROKEN PLACES*

"Quentin Vennie rose up against all odds and everyone's
expectations, including his own. In a standoff with his inner demons,
he chose a path outside of his current reality and found himself a completely
new existence, aligned with his deepest desires to rise. Quentin's raw
sharing of his incredible story inspires us to make the
changes today we want to see in our lives."

–TARA STILES, founder of Strala Yoga

"Quentin is a true phoenix. His wrenching story documents a
broken man who has been burned in so many ways, yet has refused
to be held down. His determined fight to rise from the ashes and be
born again is guaranteed to inspire and ignite inspiration in
anyone who reads it."

**–Kathryn Budig, author of *The Women's Health Big Book of Yoga*
and *Aim True***

STRONG
IN THE
BROKEN
PLACES

QUENTIN VENNIE

WITH
JON STERNFELD

RODALE.

RODALE *wellness*

Live happy. Be healthy. Get inspired.

Sign up today to get exclusive access to our authors, exclusive bonuses, and the most authoritative, useful, and cutting-edge information on health, wellness, fitness, and living your life to the fullest.

Visit us online at RodaleWellness.com
Join us at RodaleWellness.com/Join

Rodale books may be purchased for business or promotional use or for special sales. For information, please write to: Trade Books/Special Markets Department, Rodale, Inc., 733 Third Avenue, New York, NY 10017

Printed in the United States of America

Rodale Inc. makes every effort to use acid-free ♾, recycled paper ♻.

Book design by Amy King

Library of Congress Cataloging-in-Publication Data is on file with the publisher.

ISBN-13: 978-1-62336-822-7 hardcover

Distributed to the trade by Macmillan

2 4 6 8 10 9 7 5 3 1 hardcover

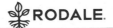

RODALE.

We inspire health, healing, happiness, and love in the world.
Starting with you.

To my mom, CHRIS, AND JAYDEN—
I HOPE I'm mAKiNG YOU PROUD.

CONTENTS

INTRODUCTION

The book you are now holding in your hands is something of a miracle. Or maybe it would be more accurate to say that it's a miracle I'm alive to write it. Considering where I was not that long ago, the fact that I'm still here—and able to tell my story—feels like a miracle to me.

Strong in the Broken Places is not a typical wellness book because I didn't live a typical wellness life. I grew up in a world where certain things were valued and others weren't, where we had access to things like liquor stores, fast food, and minimum wage jobs but were excluded from the things we really needed, like quality healthcare, financial literacy, and first-rate educations. When I faced problems, I solved them in the way I was taught: Suck it up. Stay strong. Fight back. Pain was something everyone had to deal with but no one ever talked about; you gritted your teeth and pushed through it. That's just how it was.

And it seemed to work for a long time. Until it didn't.

I stumbled across the wellness world at a moment of deep desperation. I was addicted to prescription medication and was drinking too much. I was depressed, with no faith that I could break the downward spiral I was trapped in. It was a completely random turn of events that put yoga, meditation, and juicing in my path, but it is no exaggeration to say that they saved my life.

Out of desperation, I reached for something that could lift me up and give me the strength to be a new person. This is the story of what I found and how it impacted my life in a sudden and powerful way. This book doesn't offer a traditional path to healing or wellness because that's not the one I took—I had to create my own.

As a black man raised in an impoverished neighborhood by a single mother, I was not exposed to even the most basic forms of health and wellness. For me and my mother, survival had a decidedly different connotation. For many people who grew up like I did, wellness is viewed as a luxury—something to maybe embark upon once the bills were paid or during a free Saturday, if they had one. But that's not true at all; it was my commitment to being a healthy person—inside and out—that brought me back from the brink.

The sad fact is that communities like the one I grew up in could benefit the most from having exposure to the power of wellness, whether through diet, exercise, yoga, or meditation. Growing up in my community, wellness was not a thing I saw in my neighborhood. It was not instilled in me by my parents, and it wasn't encouraged by my peers. It wasn't on any of our radars.

Wellness tools of all kinds are seldom available in the communities that need it most. My goal is to shed light on how society neglects the people and communities that need wellness initiatives, while providing them with something they were never given—not just access, but a reflection of themselves: someone just like them who went through it. I had to take charge on my own, discover the tools for myself, and apply them to my life without any sense of where I was going or whether I'd make it.

I'm a person of faith, and I don't hesitate to say that it was divine intervention that saved me, delivering these tools when I needed them to keep myself breathing. My mission is now in spreading that healing power, working to bring yoga, meditation, and other wellness tools to underserved communities. The forgotten neighborhoods and populations need it more than anyone, yet they are the ones who have the least access. I'm trying to do my part to change that.

There are some fantastic books out there for readers looking to embark on the journey of wellness, but there are virtually no books that approach health and healing from a perspective like mine. I know because I looked for them when I needed them the most.

I'm hoping to fill that gap. To tell the story of healing from a perspective of an outsider who had the need, but didn't see the way out. Not until right before the train was about to hit me.

Though I hope my story can offer some inspiration or assistance, this book is not a guide. It is my personal story. I can only hope that its very existence is a thing of value.

PART I

CHILD'S POSE

Train up a child in the way he should go: and
when he is old, he will not depart from it.

PROVERBS 22:6

CHILD'S POSE IS A RESTFUL POSE. It's often used in the beginning or middle of *asana*, the physical practice of yoga. Considered a
foundation pose, it helps to establish a conscious awareness of the
breath, as well as movement from the core. It helps to cultivate the
patience needed to surrender to the idea of nothingness while broaden-
ing awareness of the world around you.

CHAPTER

1

RESIDUE

I AM 10 YEARS OLD AND SOMETHING HAS WOKEN me up.

I'm in bed at my grandparents' house in West Baltimore, staring at the ceiling fan. It's whirring and humming in the morning din. The child in me wants to jump up and start yelling into it, get that muffled robotic drone going.

The clock radio is a red 5:05. I sense the reason I'm awake before I actually hear it. Noise is leaking in from downstairs. Muted objects shifting around the linoleum floor, voices rising and falling. Nothing concrete enough to make out, but something is clearly going on.

It's the story of my young life: reality intruding on my inner world, demanding an audience, while I try to block it out.

I peer over in bed and notice Uncle Jason is gone. This is his room, his bed. Jason is only 2 years older than me, more like a brother to me than to my father. Pop has been a ghost these days; I haven't seen him for weeks—maybe months—and the last time was for about 30 seconds.

My eyes drift outside, past the paint-chipped window frame, out to the green roof of St. Ambrose Church. I replay my latest moves on the church's basketball court, how I blew by that scrawny kid, breaking his ankles with my crossover. I've never been tall—I'll never be tall, they say—but I'm quicker than everyone else.

Grandma's house has always been a safe place, but it's an island in the middle of one of America's most dangerous cities. The noise could be an intruder, some junkie scouring for a few bucks. Or someone's broken in through the back door to grab the television. Maybe he's tossing things, taking any valuable he can find. Jason could be scuffling with him in the living room, and the guy could be going for his gun. The noise settles and then drops.

It's quiet again.

People call me Juice. My grandmother says it's because as a baby, I had juicy lips from drooling all the time. But my name is Quentin, which I hate.

My mom and I live in the Baltimore suburbs—what everyone calls "the county"—but I spend just about every weekend, summer, and break here at my father's parents' house in Park Heights. I love the comforting routine here, waking up to breakfast with my grandmother and uncle.

"Juice, you want one piece of fried bologna or two?" my grandmother would ask.

"Two," I'd say. Fried bologna's my favorite, so I'm always trying to score some extra.

"Eggs and scrapple too, right?"

"Yes, please."

"Hand me that loaf of bread in there," she'd say, head jutting to the old breadbox. Then she'd give me a cup of coffee. "And take this upstairs to your grandfather before he has a fit." That was every Saturday morning.

Except this one.

A voice pushes up through the floor, like a jolt. I don't know what's happening downstairs and I'm too afraid to find out. I just want to go back to sleep: where I feel safest, where nothing is real, where I can be whomever I want.

I close my eyes, but my mind doesn't rest. Something's whispering, nudging me to find out what's happening downstairs. I'm after answers.

I open my eyes again, or maybe they open on their own.

The noise downstairs lifts—furniture shifting, bursts of yelling, but I don't move. I stick my finger into the hole in the lining of the comforter, see how far it can go. I look outside and watch the clouds float lazily behind the church. This is my defense: *Separate yourself.* It's how I once stayed protected from my parents' fighting; now I do it all the time, avoiding loud noises and crowded places. I like it all stripped bare, down to the basics. No surprises that way.

I've seen enough of this neighborhood, out with Pop on the streets near addicts lining up to get their fix. People sleeping wherever, snorting or shooting whatever, willing to do whatever to make it through the day. Bad shit building up like a dam that could burst at any second. Spill right into Grandma's house.

I'm scared, but I have a growing sense of duty, especially to my family.

I throw the covers off and dart out of bed, hoping the momentum will bring courage. I take the stairs two at a time—trying to outrun my anxiety—and smack right into the arm of my grandmother's emerald green sofa, wrapped in thick plastic. I get up and trip over the rug runner that stretches from the front door to the dining room. I gather myself again and run toward the noise—through the empty dining room, the narrow kitchen, and down the wooden stairs to the basement.

I run around my grandfather's pool table, past his poster of sex positions on the wall, all the way to the bar in the back. At the far wall I see Uncle Jason kneeling down in front of the pullout bed. Just seeing him makes me relax. I exhale. There are no strangers around; no one is struggling, no one is fighting. Everything is frozen still when I walk in, like a painting. Just Jason. And my grandmother in the back room by the washing machine, gone quiet for a moment.

Jason is holding a small mirror with a powdered residue smeared across it. I'm not sure what it is, but I know it's not baby powder.

"Yo, what's that?" I ask him, still out of breath. "What's going on?"

Jason looks up. He's never been one to sugarcoat things for me. "Puddin' gone off that dope, yo."

Puddin' is my father's childhood nickname, though I call him Pop. "Gone off" means hooked. Dope is heroin.

My father had spread drugs on the mirror, using the hard surface to separate the powder into lines, making sure he didn't waste any and making it easier to sniff. The powder is the residue of the heroin he had snorted—a few hours earlier, right below all of us.

That discovery was the dividing line of my childhood. It was like a screeching halt and then a sharp right turn. And that morning felt like one long skid out. Even with my habit of disappearing inside myself, I couldn't ignore the truth anymore: My father was a drug addict. For a long time my family wanted to protect me from it, afraid of what I would think of him if I knew.

"I can't believe he did this shit in my house!" my grandmother was yelling from the back of the basement. "In my house! Doing this shit in my house!"

Grandma, Pop's mother, looked out for my father the most. She fed him, housed him, gave him money; everything his life was built on had come from her. But Granddad knew what being a drug addict meant. "They're thieves," he had said. "Do whatever it takes to get that hit. Only a matter of time before he steals from us." But my grandmother was not willing to turn her back on her son.

"I can't believe he'd go and do this shit in my house," she was saying. "I can't fucking believe him!"

"What do we do?" Jason asked, seemingly to me.

"—in my house!" Grandma's voice was rising again, swirling on repeat.

"I didn't even know he was here last night," Jason continued.

My heart dropped. "Wait, last night? He was here last night?" I said.

"Yeah, Mommy let him in," Jason said.

I was more in shock that my father had just been there—and that I didn't know about it—than about what he had left behind.

It cut right through me. My 10-year-old brain went into overdrive while the family around me collapsed. My father, whom I rarely saw, had snuck into the house where I was sleeping to get his fix and then vanished with the morning light. I felt like the residue, left over and forgotten.

Jason got up off of the one knee. "I knew something was up," he said, "but I ain't know he was gone like that. Ain't no coming back now." Jason was barely 12 years old, but had already seen more than people twice his age. He seemed grown to me, practically a man. I took his words as gospel. *Ain't no coming back now.*

Jason told me that Pop had called my grandmother and said he needed a place to sleep for the night. Grandma said he could stay in the basement—he'd be on the street otherwise—but he had to be gone in the morning before my grandfather woke up.

For years, all the signs of my father's addiction were there: He was too skinny, never kept promises, had trouble with the cops, couldn't hold a job, always asked for money. An addict. Just the word itself was too heavy to say. I didn't want to admit it to myself. What kid would?

Earlier that year, my father had been arrested, the first of what would become a pattern of events over the next few years. My mother explained to me that he had a few "issues" that he needed to work out, and that jail would help him. His world had been slowly killing him, and some time away would do him good. I didn't know much, but I knew what kind of friends he had. I had met them.

Jason and I would be waiting our turn for flavored ices at the snow-ball stand, and addicts would be lined up behind the Chinese carryout, waiting to receive tester pills of whatever new drug had just hit the streets. That place was a hub for drug activity, which meant it was a magnet for a lot of other things, including guns and violence. As one of the only businesses open on that strip, it was also the hangout spot we'd use for shelter from the summer heat, or the place we'd run into when-ever the police would sweep in just to harass people.

Pop would sometimes take me out and introduce me around. "Y'all know this is my son, right?" he'd say proudly, his scrawny arm around me, presenting me like a trophy. I'd force a smile. Pop was no longer the clean-cut, polished gentleman from old photographs. Hair unkempt, clothes frayed, the same gray sweatpants he always wore, large enough for us both to climb inside. These other men—I knew what they were doing. I just couldn't yet build that bridge from them to Pop.

Knowledge of my father's addiction had always been secondhand, something I never looked at directly. I was protected from it, but I also had an adolescent brain that couldn't piece things together—or didn't want to. I had seen his addiction reflected in things—his behavior, his arrests, his treatment of others, his absences. But that morning at my grandmother's house was a harsh look right at it. Like staring at the sun.

"Maybe I can talk to him," I said to Jason. "I can get him to stop whatever he's doing. I'm his son, right?" I wanted the love a father has for his son to be stronger than the pull of any addiction. Maybe if I had the opportunity to tell him how much he meant to me, he would stop using. Maybe he'd become the father I needed him to be. Hearing me, my grandmother came out from the back room. The look on her face said it all.

Even at 10, I knew this was magical thinking on my part. But I wanted to matter, to have the power to inspire Pop to turn his life around. I was already an insecure kid. Now I felt lied to, abandoned, and disowned by the one man who was supposed to love and protect me. Maybe my expectations were too high, or maybe we had different interpretations of what our relationship was supposed to be. But that morning, over that mirror, it all crumbled.

A switch was flipped in my young brain. I stopped trusting, stopped believing in people. I refused to believe in anything but disappointment. I vowed to never allow anyone to hurt me as badly as my father had, to never show how much I cared. I promised myself to be as cold and heartless to others as the world had been to me. I would show nothing: I'd be all sword, all shield.

CHAPTER
2

SURVIVAL
IN BALTIMORE

I HAVE VERY FEW PICTURES FROM MY YOUTH. The house in the first picture on the opposite page caught fire a few years later. We pulled up to see it engulfed in flames. Ma left me out front and tried to run in to rescue what she could, but the firefighters blocked her at the door. We didn't have many valuables, but what we did have—toys, baby pictures, some home movies—was destroyed. It was like my past also went up in smoke.

The picture is from my second birthday, during the time when Ma and I were moving around a lot. The house was a relative's, where my mother and I were living at the time. Ma's youngest brother, Chuck, is

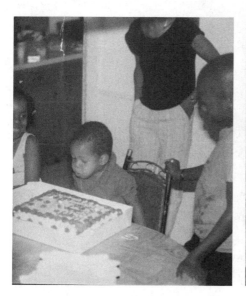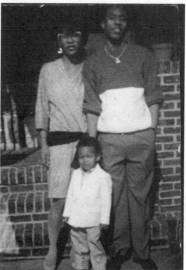

standing on the right. My mother and her tight-knit family tried to provide a sense of normalcy that I'd forever be chasing.

The second picture is the only one I know of that shows me as a child with both of my parents. It was taken on a Sunday morning, before or after church. The brick steps are in front of my grandmother's house, which I'd visit every weekend. I recognize that flashy smile on my father's face. Pop was clean, sober, and vibrant, not yet dragged down by the addiction that would come to define him. We look like a family. That's what tears at me when I look at the picture now. There's a heavy sadness because the image is a perpetual *what-if* staring back at me. It encompasses what could've been and what I wish would've been. I see the innocent child I am, unaware of how bad things were and how much worse they were going to become.

I was almost 2 years old the first time my mother broke free of my father. He left to work the overnight shift at his job and she snatched me up, grabbed a bag and a couple bottles of milk, and took off in the middle of the night. It was 2 a.m. and she was walking up Park Heights Avenue, one of the most dangerous streets in Baltimore, trying to hail a cab to get a ride to a friend's apartment.

My mother and father had first met at the KFC across the railroad tracks from my grandmother's house, and their volatile relationship, from what I've heard, was there from the word go. My father was very jealous and extremely argumentative, always assuming my mother was dealing with other guys behind his back, which she denied. His jealousy, mixed with his explosive attitude, led to frequent verbal abuse directed at my mother. She felt trapped and desperately needed to get out. Not only did she fear for her safety, but she was concerned about me growing up in such a destructive household.

After she left, the mother of one of her friends took us in. I was going to preschool at the time and my mother was working two full-time jobs, struggling to make ends meet. We'd flip-flop between the houses of her brother, sisters, and father just so we wouldn't wear out our welcome.

For the next few years, we lived anywhere we were accepted, with different relatives and friends all over Baltimore City. I have memories of staying with different uncles and aunts, sharing rooms and splitting beds with different cousins. I remember weekends at my grandparents' house, buying a plastic swimming pool at the dollar store and filling it up from a hose in the cement backyard. Grandma would throw candy in there and the local kids and I would dunk our heads in to grab what we could. It was pure, undistilled joy—blindly flailing for candy, laughing as water spouted and dripped. Jason would take me to the park and teach me how to throw and catch a football—things that fathers usually did.

Though she grew up around poverty and addiction, Ma always knew that life could, and should, be better. She worked two or three jobs at a time to get me out of Baltimore City. By the time I turned 5, she had saved up enough money to pull us over the county line. The timing was intentional; elementary school in the county required a county address.

I was part of a wave of city kids in the late 1980s who snatched county addresses like the golden tickets they were. My mother knew what was at stake with the right zip code—it was like wings.

Ma was solid, but not unmovable. She granted me a long leash, letting me veer out and make mistakes on my own. But she made sure that when it all came crashing down, she was there to help build it back up. She had a nurturing, compassionate side, but she had to be a father as well, and tried to toughen me up.

My county elementary school was only about 15 minutes from my grandmother's house in the city, but those miles covered universes. The school was in an Orthodox Jewish neighborhood; on the clean sidewalks that cut through freshly cut grass, I'd see packs of Jewish men with long beards and black hats. They traveled in unison, carrying a sense of community like an aura that trailed them down the street. They had their own stores with their own food—Kosher crackers and Manischewitz wine. It was all baffling, a total mystery to me.

School was filled mostly with white kids from freestanding houses who still lived with both of their parents. There was a calm around town—when I went into the stores or traversed parking lots, it was quiet and relaxing. None of the impending danger I was used to. None of the off-the-rails feeling that defined life in the city.

Out in the county, I learned quickly how different I was. I had to learn how to function in this new world, who I would be, and, eventually, what I thought they would let me be. My roots grew from a different place, and I was a product of history that was beyond my control. For one thing, alcohol and addiction ran on both sides of my family. When we'd visit my mom's aunts and uncles, they'd always be drinking—beer, malt liquor, harder stuff—at all hours of the day. They were a loud and abrasive bunch. One of my mom's aunts was once cursing up a storm right in front of me, and my mom turned to her and asked, "Do you have to use so many curses?"

"If you don't want his motherfucking ass to hear what I'm motherfucking saying," she said, "then cover his motherfucking ears."

That was my normality. Kids can adjust to just about anything, and I felt more comfortable back in the city than I did at school. It's also where my heart was. On Fridays when school let out, I'd finish my homework and take off for Park Heights and Wiley Avenue to hang out with Jason and my friends from the old neighborhood. Addicts and drug dealers were always around, but I knew the core of those people. I didn't look at them as derelicts or bottom feeders—I still don't. They're just people. I grew up surrounded by what my county neighbors might think is a horror, things and people they would cross the street to avoid. But these were my neighbors, my friends and family. When they're a part of you, labels aren't so easily slapped on.

Mom and I floated in that purgatory for years, never far enough away to be safe. In fact, Baltimore County is where a lot of the drug dealers lived. They would do their work in the city but wanted a safe haven from the drama, a quiet place to rest their heads and raise their children. Even drug dealers crave safer streets. But in that underworld, there is a limited separation; the same attention that paid their bills could follow them home to their front door.

I remember the first place we lived in the county, where we moved when I was 5 years old. It was a small apartment complex of faded brown brick and siding. We lived on the second floor and my mother's bedroom window faced the front of the apartment complex, looking onto the parking lot and front steps. The apartment was off Liberty Road, the main throughway connecting the city and county, the vein running through my two worlds.

Once I woke up to the sounds of a scuffle right outside my window, two men yelling followed by a loud pop, then another. Ma was in bed with me, lying down low, the television on mute. She saw me rustle and pushed me back down.

"Quentin," she whispered, "don't say nothing, don't do nothing." We laid there quiet. "Don't make a sound," she mouthed. I went stiff, frozen.

If I had lifted up my head, I could have seen it all out the window. A few minutes later a man was banging on our door, asking for help, begging for us to call the police. My mother inched low over to the living room and called 911. Then she came back, and we huddled in my twin bed. About 5 minutes later, sirens pierced the quiet night. We called my grandfather, who came by to get us. On our way out, I saw blood spattered on the door and pooling on the concrete walkway. The ambulance had just taken the guy away, and they were uncoiling the water hoses to spray down the pavement.

//

My father was only 17 when I was born, so as I grew up, he was still trying to figure out who he was. In some ways we had to grow up simultaneously, on parallel tracks. In my early years, when he was still clean, he worked as a manager at a Checkers fast-food joint. Sometimes my mom would drop me there and I'd sit at a booth and he'd bring me a free meal. When I was done, he'd take me into the back kitchen; I'd be enthralled by the deep fryers bubbling and the cooks chopping, the orders whipping through. He'd show me around, and that value made me proud. After his shift ended, I'd stay with him for the weekend, sometimes to give Ma a break, but usually because she had to work.

When I was 6, Pop's girlfriend gave birth to my half-sister, Nicole, and that was when the change came over him. My sister's birth seemed to give him an excuse to ignore me. When I visited his apartment, he'd seem irritated I was there, complaining that he couldn't "get a break." I'd want to spend time together—just watch television or help him cook—and he would get annoyed. Pop wasn't the most patient person, but he was also young and stuck at home with a baby most of the time; when the weekend would come around and he'd be desperate for a break, I would show up.

Sometimes I was witness to my father's violence; other times I was the target. One incident is carved into my brain. I was staying with him for the weekend and his girlfriend had taken the baby to her mother's, so it was just the two of us. Pop's go-to meal was spaghetti, and he could cook the hell out of it as far as I was concerned. We sat down to eat and I must've scarfed down my bowl in 2 minutes. Like most kids, my eyes were bigger than my stomach.

"Can I have some more?" I asked. "Please?"

He looked up, almost suspicious. "All right, Quentin, but if I give you some more, you better eat it."

"No problem. I'ma eat it." He piled it high on my plate, thick and steaming. I saw him watching me tight as I struggled through that second helping, like he was waiting to jump. A few bites in, my stomach started to shut down. I was stuffed. I dropped my fork, and with that light clang, his eyes darted up to me across the table.

"Uh-uh, Quentin," he said. "You're gonna eat that."

"But I'm full!"

He threw his fork down. "I don't care. You're not getting up from this table until you finish it. You're not gonna waste food in my house."

"What? What am I supposed to do?"

"You're gonna sit there and finish it." He got up to bring his empty plate to the sink in the kitchen.

I just sat there in my stubbornness. "Okay," I yelled. "I'll just be here all night until Ma comes to pick me up!"

There was silence, then the sound of him breathing in. I heard the hard rattle of the dish hitting the metal sink. Then Pop was on me. He grabbed me out of the chair by my shirt, threw my 40 pounds across the room. I tripped on the table leg and landed on the hardwood in the living room. Then he came at me, bull-like, and picked me up again. He dragged me through the apartment to the bedroom, me kicking and flailing, him dogged and scary. As we crossed into the bedroom, Pop lifted me up and tossed me onto the bed with such force that I bounced off the mattress and landed on the floor. By this point, I was hysterically crying.

In his mind I was being disobedient, talking back and showing disrespect. That could've been what triggered it. Or maybe it had nothing to do with me.

"You're staying in here for the rest of night!" he railed. "Don't come out until your mother comes to get you." He slammed the door, setting me off on another crying spurt.

I had seen this side of Pop before, but I was overwhelmed that it was being directed toward me. It was confusing: I loved my father, but I was terrified of him. I cried silently, jamming my head into a pillow to muffle the noise, afraid of what would happen if he came back. The clock froze as I tried to figure out how long until my mother would come and get me. I wanted to tell her what happened, but I knew there would then be a fight between my parents and she wouldn't allow me back there for a while. Or maybe I didn't want to come back. With my face stuffed in that pillow, I just wanted to go home, crawl into bed, and go to sleep, surrounded in the safe shell once again. A place where no one could touch me.

About an hour later, I heard voices and rumblings. People in the apartment. "Get yourself together," my father popped in and said. "Your grandparents and uncle are here."

"I don't care!" I yelled. "I want to go home. I'm not leaving till Ma gets here!"

"Shh," he said, trying to calm me down. He closed the door behind him. "Don't say anything. Calm down. Look, I'm gonna put on *Thriller* and you get out there and do some Michael Jackson for everyone." It was more of a demand than an offer. "Get yourself together and come out."

I worshipped Michael Jackson, and I would imitate him any chance I got. I used to beg my mother for a Michael Jackson wig, white glove, and red leather jacket like from the "Thriller" video. She told me we didn't need them—I didn't understand the concept of poor—so I'd dress up with what I could piece together and put on a show. I was really into break dancing at the time—that free-flowing energy, the electricity buzzing through my body. It made me feel alive, gave me presence, a slight sense of magic and power. I'd watch the *Breakin'* movies and practice along with Ozone's moves: the sidestep, the pop and lock, the float, the freeze. And I could do Michael step for step: the circle slide, the hip thrust, the spin, and, of course, the moonwalk.

My grandparents especially loved this routine and Pop didn't give me much choice in the matter. I walked out of the room, reluctant at first. I could tell we were engaging in a different kind of performance as well—the typical father-son weekend, the happy family.

When I got out, my father dropped the needle on "Billie Jean"—the hi-hat, then the bass, then the synthesizer line—woom, *woom, woom,* woom—and I was transformed, channeling my idol across the living room's hardwood floor.

Pop was presenting normalcy, covering up the fact that he had gotten so mad over something so small. My grandmother knew how he was, was well aware of why his relationship with my mother imploded: his attitude, his anger, and his jealousy, which would rise up like a monster from inside of him. He was still a young man, and he didn't want to hear his mother's reprimands. As for me, I jumped at the chance to perform—to be the center for once. It was easy. We both just painted it all over.

As I made my way through elementary school, Pop began to fade. The visits became less regular, then spotty, then canceled with no explanation.

A typical scenario: One Friday afternoon at my mom's house, the phone rang.

"Hey, Quentin," my father said, channeling his old self, energized and charming. "I'm on my way to come to pick you up. Make sure you have your clothes and be ready."

Excited, I started to pack, shoving clothes into a bag for the weekend, carefully picking out which toys I'd bring: He-Man and Skeletor, Sgt. Slaughter and Hulk Hogan with a black marker circle around his eye, broken GI Joes my cousins gave to me. I tucked my He-Man blanket under my arm and took one last look around to make sure I had everything.

"Quenti-i-i-i-in!" my mom yelled from the kitchen. "Come out, your father will be here soon!"

"Coming!"

"Just wait in here," my mom said when I came out. "You'll hear him."

"Nah, I'll wait outside." My anticipation took over, running through me like a wire.

"Okay," she said, "but come in if it's too long. It's cold out there."

I walked down the apartment steps and sat at the bottom, waiting to spot that gold Toyota Corolla rounding the corner. I replayed my last visit and what I might've done to make him mad; how I'd be better this weekend; how maybe he'd take me out to meet his friends; how because my sister was getting older, maybe there'd be less stress around his house. I was oblivious as to why Pop had changed; like most kids, I blamed myself.

Ten minutes passed. Then another 10.

"Come back in the house," my mom yelled through our third-floor window. "I'll page him and see where he is. You can go back out when he's closer."

"Nah, I'll wait out here." I thought that maybe if I stayed there, he would come. Like I could will it to happen. Like if I was already out there, the visit had already started and he would have to show.

Thirty minutes. Forty minutes. I kept waiting, but it was obvious he wasn't coming. I started crying, and Ma called through the window.

"He's not coming, Q. I'm sorry. Come back into the house."

And I did, sullen and drained.

I remember those times in a progression, an accordion opening outward. The first few times that my father let me down, she broke it gently and tried to comfort me. "It's going to be okay," she'd say. "You got me. Everything's going to be all right." And I got accustomed to her compassion. I wanted her to hold me and tell me it was going to be all right.

But after enough of those Fridays, a switch flipped. She refused to let me wallow. If I cried, she'd try to spike it. "Straighten yourself up," she'd say. "That's his loss. You're not gonna cry over this man." Or, "Suck it up, Q. You gotta deal with it."

It felt cruel at the time but I'm a parent now, and I understand what she was trying to teach me: This could go on your whole life, so you might as well acclimate to it. It was protection and preparation for a certain kind of life and a certain kind of father. But there was an unintended consequence. The lesson I took away from it was that I didn't have the right to feel.

Where I grew up, there's a code that you have to repress and hide, put on a tough shell, or else put yourself at risk. So that opening, that release valve, that permission to feel got closed up inside of me. And the pressure bled into other things. I didn't have an outlet to ask for help, didn't even feel allowed to seek one, so I felt trapped. That feeling thickened as I got older. The seeds of later issues and addictions were planted there, in that bottling process.

"Mom, that's just wrong," I'd say. "That's not fair."

"Well, that's how the world is," she'd respond. "Everything in this world is not going to be built the way you want it to be."

Coming from where we did, we didn't see a lot of justice. Teachers, parents, police—no one seemed to act the way they were supposed to. "I'm preparing you for survival in the city of Baltimore," Ma would say. I wanted justice, but my mother was interested in the reality of living. She taught me to show a warrior to the world, one who refused to be taken down. Whether I felt like one was beside the point.

I was always insular and forced to adapt to what I was given. As an only child who moved around a lot and had few friends, I spent a lot of time playing by myself. It gave me an observer's perch, the time and distance to put people together. I was obsessed with logic, wanted everything to make sense, to fit—and it killed me that it didn't. The discrepancy between what was and what I thought should be was massive. Trying to exist in that space would become my defining struggle.

CHAPTER
3

THE CURTAIN

AS MY FATHER FADED FROM MY LIFE, I blamed myself, thinking I was the thing he wanted to escape from. The worst part was that he wasn't even really gone; sometimes he was hiding in plain sight. One Saturday morning I was heading with Jason up to Lucille's, a park with one of the few open basketball courts in my grandmother's neighborhood, practicing my crossover on the sidewalk. That court was next to a liquor store and steps away from one of the area's biggest heroin corners. My uncle and I knew the dealer, so we were always safe, but I was still on guard.

Jason elbowed me, gesturing forward and shaking his head. I looked up ahead and saw a bony figure, scarecrow thin. His clothes were draped loosely as if on a hanger. It was my father, leaning against a rickety fence, though it was more like the fence was holding him up.

He was nodding off, in and out of consciousness, too high to notice me. As we passed him, I saw his skin was ashen, his heavy eyes shut. It was painful, being so close but not being seen, within reach but not being able to touch.

I also felt shame: He was out in the open, and the two of us were one—I was his son, my name was his, and here he was for everyone to see. Other times, riding through the old neighborhood with my mother, I'd catch quick glimpses of him on the sidewalk or on corners. Pop would be right there through the car window, on the other side of the glass, but miles away. He'd become a vision, a flicker on a television screen, a ghost.

On weekends when Pop would drop in at my grandparents' house, desperation hovered around him like a cloud; he was dirty and worn down, his skin hanging like an old man's. He would silently devour a plate of food, veiny eyes straining toward some invisible point in the distance. He'd get up, collect some cash from my grandmother, and be gone before I could say goodbye. Then he'd disappear for weeks at a time. I started to think it'd be easier if I didn't know him at all. At least I wouldn't feel that gap, that giant hole. I reasoned that I couldn't miss something that I never had. I'd said this to my mother more than once. "You don't mean that," she'd say. But I wasn't so sure. My father's addiction was a pain that kept revisiting, leaving fresh scars each time.

I didn't understand at the time that Pop was an addict, doing what addicts do. He was having run-ins with the police—mostly for drugs, once for stealing his girlfriend's car. Things escalated in tandem: I was getting old enough to notice things and Pop's life was spiraling at a faster clip. We were headed on a collision course, hurtling toward impact. His reality would inevitably shatter into mine.

When I was 9—about a year before the heroin discovery in my grandmother's basement—the curtain covering his world inched open. One night, Pop took me and my sister Nicole, who was 3, to the movies to see

Home Alone 2. It was a comedy about a family struggling to put itself back together, the problems all solvable, the hurdles hilarious. Clear heroes, obvious villains. It was pure fantasy, and I loved it. After the movie, we caught a hack cab back to my grandmother's house.

"Go on in the house," Pop told us as we pulled up. "I'll see y'all tomorrow. I got some things to take care of." I grabbed Nicole's hand as we crossed the busy road and headed inside. When I turned to wave goodbye, he was gone.

My grandmother woke me early the next morning, frantic. "Juice, put your clothes on! Juice! Get up! We gotta go to Maude's house." Maude was her mother, who lived on Poplar Grove in a rough area of West Baltimore. I came to life against the dawn. "What's going on?" I asked.

"Something's happened to your father," she yelled back to me, hustling down the stairs.

I threw on some clothes and hurried to follow her out, my heart skittering the whole ride there. In the car, I asked a lot of questions but she just ignored me and stared ahead as she drove, elbows out, fingers gripped tight. I could see fear in her eyes, a panic rising up on her face. We pulled up to Maude's, her block a row of faded red brick row houses and slivered patches of high grass. The neighborhood was silent except for a barking dog, a few morning drinkers, and a bus carrying some early shifters. As we entered, the door creaked, cutting through the silent house. Grandma took my hand as we walked up the three flights of stairs. At the top we entered a small dark room with red wallpaper, a room that had always spooked me. All the kids usually stayed away from it, like it was haunted.

My father was lying there on a thin bed, almost unrecognizable. His body was limp, his face swollen and bloody. There was an awful smell in there, like the lingering scent of death. Pop was holding a washcloth wrapped around ice up to his face, trying to bring the swelling down. My grandmother ran up to him. "What happened, what happened, what happened?!" she kept asking. But he wouldn't speak. He just laid there, silently staring at a small television on mute. Dried tears shone on his weathered face. He was clearly in pain, but there was also this wounded pride. Pop had a reputation as a fighter, and he had been a respected presence in the area. He seemed shocked that someone had gotten to him.

The whole experience felt fragmented to me, the emotions easier to access than the facts. Pop finally turned to my grandmother and whispered. I couldn't hear him, but I saw the panic on her face. "Listen, don't do nothing stupid," my grandmother told him. "You don't want to get yourself locked up again. It's not worth it. Let it be."

"Yeah, don't do anything," I said. "It's not worth it. We just went to the movies yesterday. That was fun, wasn't it?" I was still naive enough to think that our bond could somehow save him.

He didn't respond, wouldn't even let his eyes meet mine. I was trying to stay strong, to show him that I was tough enough to handle this. But I couldn't take it. Any of it.

After about 15 minutes in there, I walked down the narrow hallway to the bathroom and sat on the cold floor, my back up against the closed door. I started crying into my sleeve and I could not stop. I leaned forward and flushed the toilet a few times to skirt any suspicion. Once I felt like I had emptied myself out, I stood up: a deep inhale, a putting back on of the armor. *Get it together, Quentin.* I splashed some water on my face and walked back into that room. Maude was in there now; she and my grandmother were silent, Maude lightly brushing Pop's hair, my grandmother holding his hand. I stayed in the doorway.

Pop was too stubborn to go to the hospital. He just laid there resigned, bleeding all over his clothes, the sheets, and the pillows. Then his head turned, as if a rope slowly yanked him. "Go home, Ma," he said. "Just . . . go home."

My grandmother froze, like she'd been cut. Maybe she was thinking about how my grandfather might've been right, that giving up was the only way.

"Okay," she said, "but don't call me to bail your fucking ass out of jail for this dumb shit. Your ass is alive and that should be enough."

She walked out of the room and stormed downstairs, mumbling something under her breath. "Come on, Juice, let's go," she called back. I took one last look at my father. I wanted to hug him, maybe even give him a kiss on his forehead, just to show him that I loved him. But I couldn't bring myself to do something so out of character for either of us.

"Later, Pop," I said. He didn't move his eyes from the television. His lifelessness terrified me.

Every kid wants to feel like their father is invincible, an unshakeable force, and I was no different. That morning, seeing him so vulnerable, a discarded object, was too much. It shook the balance and left me unmoored. I left Maude's house understanding that my father lived in a much darker world than I had imagined, one that had nothing to do with movies.

At the time, everyone decided to concoct a story about what happened to keep me in the dark. I didn't find out until later what really happened: My father was a known thief around Park Heights and Poplar Grove. He and his friend had a hustle where one would create a diversion and the other would rob a drug dealer's stash house; they'd snatch the supply, then use some and sell some. The night before, after dropping my sister and me off, Pop got caught. Some guys chased him for about four blocks, grabbed him as he was running into Maude's house, and dragged him down the cement steps. They beat him with a baseball bat and cracked bottles over his head. They punched with their fists and kicked with their boots, sending a message through his face and body. If Maude's neighbor hadn't called the police, he likely would've been beaten to death.

That moment, and that memory, sliced like a blade through my whole perception of my father. Seeing him in that condition was a turning point for me, and it put a clear frame on what world he lived in. Things didn't stay inside that dark room in Maude's house—not for my father, not for any of us. My father's addiction was a flood, seeping into other parts of my world. As I made my way through elementary school,

I became defensive and angry. I was a trip wire just waiting to get triggered. At the time it didn't feel connected, but in hindsight, the link between my father and this new me was a solid, inexorable line. My fuse got shorter, and it burned lightning fast when I felt I was treated unfairly. I kept to myself until I felt someone stepped over the line. Then, without warning, I'd pounce. "Don't let anyone pick on you," my father taught me—the one piece of advice from him that I took.

\\

School was such a disconnected place that it might as well have been an alien planet. On the ride home from school, I'd see manicured lawns framing enormous houses and fences surrounding pristine playgrounds. Other kids' parents went on field trips and showed up at assemblies. The gap between them and me was a chasm. I was one of the only kids in my elementary school on the free and reduced lunch program, another mark on me. I carried a card that I'd swipe in the cafeteria that couldn't be used for snacks or candy—it was like I was policed for being poor. Two kids always bullied me in there, cutting in front of me on the lunch line, taking my milk or orange juice, hassling me. One time I calmly put down my tray and sprang: I grabbed a fistful of one of their shirts and slammed its owner back against the cinder block wall. The kid's eyes popped, stunned; he was so used to me not reacting. His friend took off running to get a teacher. I was the only one who got into trouble, but at least they left me alone after that.

In fourth grade, a new black student named Kenneth joined Mr. Redmond's class. Kenneth, with off-brand clothes and a body-odor problem, had a rough time. Other kids would walk by pinching their noses, then bust out laughing. One day Kenneth came to school transformed: fresh haircut, a blue denim jumper with suspenders. He'd redesigned himself and became fashionable and fly, accepted by the other kids. He joined them at their lunch table, and they traded jokes all through class. Once nestled comfortably in the cool group, Kenneth started to piss outside the tent. He started to taunt the only other black kid—me—trying to put more distance between the two of us.

About a week into Kenneth's torment, I snapped. I was helping some other kids clean up the classroom before dismissal at the end of the day. Kids were sweeping the floor, picking up trash, smacking together the erasers outside and creating big puffs of white. Kenneth was holding court up against his desk with two other boys, doing impressions of the other kids. I started picking up the chairs around them.

"Hey, Quentin," one of the boys said, "pick my chair up."

"No," I said. "Pick your own chair up."

He got up in my face. "You *better* pick my chair up or I'll get Kenneth to make you do it."

He thought I'd be intimidated, but I saw Kenneth for what he was: a scared boy in a mask. "You better get out of my face," I said, "'cause I'm not scared of you or Kenneth."

"You said my name?" Kenneth said, imitating what he thought tough sounded like. "You must want to do something. What you wanna do?" Kenneth was more naturally muscular than I was and started to bump his shoulder into mine. "What you gonna do?" he said with each bump. "What you gonna do?"

"I'm not in the mood, Kenneth," I said.

"I don't care what mood you're in!" he said, still bumping me, rolling his sleeves up. "You ain't gonna do nothing."

"Stop showing off," I said.

I'd exposed him, torn off his mask in front of everyone. He pushed me hard.

As he came back at me, I tucked in my chin, balled my fist, and punched him dead in the face. Everyone heard the thud—even Mr. Redmond turned around.

"I told you to stop bumping me!" I yelled.

Kenneth immediately put both his hands on his eye and started jumping up and down, screaming and crying.

"What happened?" Mr. Redmond said, cutting through the desks and chairs. "What happened here?"

"He was—" my adrenaline outpaced my words.

"He just popped Kenneth for no reason," one boy said.

"He just swung at him. We were just talking," the other boy jumped in.

"I did not!" I yelled. "He was—"

"Quentin—"

"But he was—"

"Quentin, enough! No fighting in class," Mr. Redmond said. "Get your bag and go to the office. Natalie, escort him there."

"This is bullshit!" I yelled. I snatched my bag and stormed out. Natalie walked gingerly behind me. I caught a glimpse of her and could tell she wanted to say something. She had bright green eyes, and a tooth gap that her tongue poked through. "What?"

"Nothing."

"What?!"

"I'm sure he deserved it," she said quietly. "I know you're not that kind of person."

I felt like no one knew what kind of person I really was or was capable of being. Her soft words were a small comfort at the time. I still felt as alone as I ever had.

That feeling of isolation started to harden into something like armor or a shell. My initial fear of confronting people drained away. I didn't have to accept how others treated me. There was a sense of power: *I can change this.* Some of the kids and teachers started looking at me as if I were violent, which was frustrating. I was just trying to break free of what others were trying to make me be. But all it did was box me in even more.

||||||||||||||||||||||||||||||||||||||||||||||||||||||||||||||||||||||||||||||||||||||||

Saint Bernardine Roman Catholic Church is in West Baltimore on Edmondson Avenue. It's an imposing building of gray stone with enormous and blotchy red wooden doors. White statues perch like watchmen outside a giant gold dome. The church contrasts starkly with the dilapidated row houses surrounding it—most of which were built to house the influx of families that flooded into Baltimore decades after the church was built.

Inside, the ceiling opens wide and full, revealing white walls with gold accents, cherrywood pews, color paintings of Jesus and angels in stained glass windows. A large crucifix hangs from the ceiling behind the pulpit. Some days I was dropped off at children's Bible study; other times I attended Mass with my mother, my cousin Arnita, and my mother's Aunt Brenda. I'd sit there and listen to a man in pure white drone on and on. Church was supposed to ground our hopes and desires, unite us in our fears and struggles, but none of it resonated with me. It just triggered more questions:

If God was real, why were we still struggling?

If Ma was putting her last $20 in the tithing bucket, why were we fighting to keep the lights on?

Why did God let my father become an addict, a hollow shell of his former self, wandering Park Heights Avenue?

Why were husbands and fathers lining up outside the liquor store at eight o'clock in the morning?

What was with these abandoned houses, used syringes in the gutters, empty bottles of Irish Rose on the sidewalk right outside the church? If God was so present, wouldn't he spend time right here, where he was needed the most?

Every Sunday we would seek solace and comfort at church, but to me, everyone seemed to be drawing from an empty well. The idea of praying to something I couldn't see and couldn't touch felt ridiculous. God was either not there, or not who these people thought he was. I still clung to an idea that there was something greater than us. It just seemed like we had it all wrong.

I had gotten used to straddling my two worlds—city and county—though I never quite belonged in either. In both environments I was ridiculed for being different. In school, I was known as the urban kid with the bad attitude who spoke slang and acted "ghetto." When I visited my old neighborhood, I had somehow become the county kid who spoke proper English and acted white. I was torn between two realities, embraced by neither, and privately raging inside.

Then came that fateful morning in my grandmother's basement, the heroin discovery, the new reality I had no choice but to accept: I was the son of an addict. Drugs don't just destroy one person; there's a ripple effect outward, into others' futures, careers, communities, and families. The destruction is not contained. It permeates in all directions, flooding into spaces. It's water seeking its level.

So, at 10 years old, I was looking for solace, looking for a world that could comfort and stem the flow of the pain seeping through. But I got the exact opposite. The 3 years of middle school would be a constant battle. I'd come up against an unwelcoming and cruel environment that would harden me and screw me into place.

Sudbrook was a magnet middle school, one of the most prominent in Baltimore County. At 10 years old, I underwent a college-style admissions process: a one-on-one interview with the principal, the submission of my school transcripts, a writing sample, and multiple book reports. Sudbrook had strict rules, school uniforms, and a curriculum that tried to mirror the college experience.

Sudbrook was a melting pot of cultures and ethnicities. Although white kids made up the majority of the population, there were also Asian, Hispanic, African, European, and Middle Eastern students there. Most of them came from stable two-parent households and lived in safe suburban neighborhoods stretching as far out as the upscale Reisterstown, 13 miles away. Sudbrook cast a wide net, wanting the highest-performing students so they could set the standard for what the magnet program would become. I was accepted, but never accepted. They let me in, but they never let me be.

We had to wear our khakis with either a polo shirt with SUDBROOK stitched in or an embroidered sweatshirt. The uniform felt like a lock on my free expression, so I rebelled; I wore my uniform a little baggy, as was hip-hop custom at the time. Creases weren't ironed into my khakis, and I rocked Nikes or Timberland boots instead of loafers. I tried to give the me inside that uniform some room to breathe.

I quickly got labeled as a problem kid, a derelict, an issue to be contained. It created a feedback loop where, in my frustration, I became exactly that. The label closed off who I could be, who I might have become. It forced me into a corner that I was constantly trying to wrestle out of—which of course, only made me look more unmanageable.

I got discouraged, then aggravated. None of my teachers or administrators ever inquired about who I was or where I came from. They knew nothing of my father's issues, his time in jail, my mother's struggles, and our financial stress. Teachers and administrators wrote me off as a disobedient thug, and I got boxed in. Everything I did to break free was treated as more proof that I needed the box.

When I was sent to the office—which was often—I would never go quietly. I would get up, flip my desk over, then walk out. I'd slide my chair across the room and knock the bookshelf over. I had to show I disapproved of how I was being treated, and it had to be deafening. Sudbrook was populated by multiple cultures and ethnicities, but it was dominated by upper-class white kids. I was used to looking different, but I had never been treated as so starkly separate.

I remember a classmate named Jason Williams. He was the golden boy, the All-American black kid. The class constantly got sick of hearing how we didn't measure up to Jason, who was brilliant and articulate, poised to do anything. "Why can't you black kids be more like Jason?" I'd hear. "You see how Jason is doing this?" the teachers would say. "You need to do it how Jason does it." It felt to me like white kids could be anything they wanted, but if you were black, you damn well better be like Jason Williams. No room for error. Unimpeachable.

When Jason would finish an assignment, he was given free rein. He was allowed to do other work, talk to other teachers, leave early. One time I finished my work and walked over to the bookshelf to grab the dictionary. I had read that Malcolm X studied the dictionary as a kid; he learned to cut people down with words, to the point where he was slicing up Ivy League debaters. I was also getting into music, hip-hop specifically, and was drawn to discovering new words—which were weapons in the hands of the best MCs.

"Quentin," Mrs. Stoner said, looking up from her desk. She was a short lady who always seemed to be wearing the same red sweater. "What are you doing?"

"I'm done. I was going to read the dictionary," I said, pointing at the bookshelf.

"Well, go back to your seat. You need to sit down."

"But I'm done! Jason—"

"If you're done with your work, just put your head down."

Put my head down? "What am I, five?" I said. I saw the other kids look up. "I'm not putting my head down!"

"Quentin—"

"That's not fair!" I shouted, building into a rage. "Why can Jason do things I can't?"

I was interested in logic, but I ran into a wall: Mrs. Stoner was a "because I said so" kind of person, a response that enraged me. The confrontation got me kicked out of class that day—then removed for good. For no academic reasons at all, I was put in the remedial English program. They tried to disguise it by calling it an empowering opportunity, but I knew it was the opposite. A de-fanging. I was being marginalized.

Those kinds of classes are designed to put walls around us, but they end up creating a ceiling, and a low one at that.

The remedial class was almost entirely black kids who met in the cafeteria in the morning. An African American teacher named Ms. Johnson was brought in specifically to teach us. We were assigned easy books like Robert Lipsyte's *The Contender*, stories about minority teenagers, turn-your-life-around choices, and hopeful messages. My peers were studying Shakespeare while I was being offered the only kind of character the administration thought I could relate to—young, troubled, and black. It was an insult; I wanted to be challenged. I needed my world expanded, not thrown back at me in the bleached form of a morality tale. I had earned my place in the most prestigious school in the county, and now they were taking that away from me.

"They want me to keep an eye on you guys," Ms. Johnson told us early on. She was a soft-spoken woman, gentle and kind most of the time, stern when she had to be. She wore dresses down to her feet that swooshed as she glided around the room. She held up a stack of papers and waved it around. "Here's what I'm supposed to know about you—what your teachers and counselors think I need to know." She put it down on the desk and said, "But I'm going to let you show me who you are."

This is different, I thought. I wasn't fooled simply by Ms. Johnson being black. The assistant principal was black, a mean woman with an ugly high top hairstyle, and she was even more prejudiced than the others. But Ms. Johnson cut through. She burned with light.

"I understand what you're going through, believe it or not. And between us," she leaned forward conspiratorially, "I don't agree with them. None of you belong here." She let us know that she felt what we felt, and her validation was enormous for me. I was driven by a perpetual hunt for fairness and just by calling this out, labeling it what it was, Ms. Johnson became the first adult at Sudbrook worth listening to.

I was a model student for Ms. Johnson, but in other classes I was sent to the office for everything from slapping beats on my desk to screaming out answers. Everything was always my fault. When I got into trouble, Ms. Johnson would try to speak with me prior to the principal taking over. I remember one time the principal stood waiting for me at her office door, and Ms. Johnson put her hand on my shoulder. "You know, Quentin, you're not who everyone thinks you are," she said.

I had never heard it put that way before. Her words electrified something dormant in me, something I sensed was true but had given up trying to prove. Saying it that way gave it power. Ms. Johnson saw something in me I didn't see in myself and went out of her way for me. She would walk through the halls with me, sit with me at lunch, buy me snacks if I didn't have money, and check on me in other classes.

One day, I got thrown out of one of my classes and the teacher, Mrs. Davidson, wanted me permanently moved. The next morning in the cafeteria, Ms. Johnson sat down across from me as I was eating breakfast.

"What happened yesterday?" she asked.

"When?"

"Mrs. Davidson. You know things get back to me."

"Nothing," I said, staring down at my pants. I took off my headphones and started wrapping the cord around my Walkman, the beat of Tupac's "Pain" still pushing through. "Same shit."

"You know, Quentin, I know you feel wronged. But yelling and arguing aren't getting you anywhere. Can I make a suggestion?"

"Sure."

"Why not write a letter apologizing for your reaction."

"What?!"

"Just think about it. You don't have to. But it's a good idea. This is the world—you're not always going to win. An apology might smooth things over."

Ms. Johnson knew what no one else did: I needed to be nurtured, not criticized. Because she was the first teacher who took the time to learn about me, I did as she asked. Her care was a magnet that drew out my better self.

Ms. Johnson sat across the table, looking at me like she had more to say.

"What?"

"Quentin, it's just—well, I notice you have a lot of anger in you."

This was an understatement. I was a bubbling volcano in those days.

"And you have such a way with words. If you're angry, why don't you channel that—write about how you feel." She reached into her bag and dug out a black spiral notebook, sleek and pristine. She handed it to me.

"I know you like to read the dictionary," she said, "and I know how you feel about Tupac. You know he studied poetry."

"Wait, you got this for me?"

"Yes." She smiled. "Why don't you try channeling that onto paper as opposed to, you know, just getting into trouble. Take a cue from the people you're listening to." She gestured at my Walkman. The gritty rage of Tupac's voice rumbled through into the table.

"Thanks, but I can't take this," I said. "You already do more than you're supposed to."

"Please," she insisted, "let me help you. I'm sure your mother is tired of leaving work to have to come to the principal's office. The way you're handling things, well, it's not working. Take it. See what happens."

"Thanks," I said, tucking the notebook under my arm. I walked around the table to give her a hug. Even though I pretended I couldn't accept it, I was secretly ecstatic.

CHAPTER
4

TARGET

WRITING WAS LIKE THROWING A BALL against a wall instead of launching it at other people's heads. I was still a hothead, but with a positive outlet, things were less bottled up and the venting lowered the temperature. I built my own sanctuary, a place to visit any chance I got. When I covered that first notebook, I wrote on scraps of paper and napkins and furiously scribbled on the back of my hand.

I was big into spoken word: the complexity of wordplay, the voice inflections, the fiery emotion. It provided me with an outlet to find my voice, and to express the injustice that I felt I was experiencing. Most of my poems derived from questions: "Who am I?," "Is it all worth it?," "Where do I belong?" It was my way of trying to make sense out of life, asking the question only to answer it myself on the other end. My mind never shut off—it was a churning machine, and I felt a throbbing pulse, a need to get it all down before I exploded. It kept me awake at night, half-listening to every conversation, and off task in every classroom. I started with simple rhyme patterns, syllables spaced out to a beat.

> *If my skin is a curse, then my life is a sin*
> *So I battle every day, tryin' to fight 'til I win*

Writing began as a release valve for my anger and turned into a microphone, then a bullhorn. A declaring of the me who had been fighting to get out.

As I wrote, and the thoughts flowed out, I couldn't ignore something that seemed to gird a lot of my treatment. Racism exists, I would rail, open your eyes. It wasn't a thing in books; it was happening right there in that school. The newspaper headlines opened it up; socially conscious movies such as *Do the Right Thing* and *Boyz n the Hood* made it plain. Malcolm X's autobiography and Martin Luther King Jr.'s speeches sold me on the revolutionary mind-set. It all combined for me, stewed together into a raging fire.

Ms. Johnson introduced me to poetry, gave me printouts with poems by Langston Hughes and Amiri Baraka, and let me borrow some books she brought in from home. These writers became the light that peeked through from that world—and I tried to pry the door open. I was fascinated by how the writers wielded words, used sounds as tools, how they pushed them together, let them wrestle, played them off each other. Their voices crackled with energy, purpose, and emotion. Writing began as a solitary experience, but a new self emerged from the other end. I won a few poetry contests at school and Ms. Johnson even submitted one of my poems to be featured in an anthology. I was putting my true self out there in a way that I never would have before; that kind of confidence pushed up the ceiling and broadened the walls. It was a declaration: I am somebody. I am Quentin. I am.

Later that year I heard a song by the rapper Nas, "The World Is Yours." The first verse alone was a breakthrough. It exploded my world open.

I sip the Dom P, watching Gandhi til I'm charged
*Then writing in my book of rhymes, all the words past the margin**

Nas turned the outside world into a canvas and splashed his inner monologue like paint—loud and bold and impossible to ignore. It was a revelation. I was born on the other side of those speakers.

For my 13th birthday, my friend Robert gave me Jay-Z's first album, *Reasonable Doubt*. It became a flashpoint. I wore that CD out in my scratched-up silver Discman. My favorite way to listen was cocoon mode: I'd go to my room, close the door, and sit on the floor with my back against my bed. I'd put on those plastic headphones, close my eyes, drop my head, and zone in. It was all about shutting the world out—and making room for this new one.

Jay-Z came from a rough neighborhood and had witnessed the same pain and turmoil I carried with me as both a badge and a chain. Jay was a smart kid who was rejected from mainstream society, written off as a problem, unaware of his potential. His father was a drug addict who was absent from his life; his mother struggled to get him through. In my bedroom, I'd immerse myself in his baritone street voice, standing on the corner with him, fighting his fights, carrying his weight. His story was a version of mine that I could understand.

On tracks such as "Dead Presidents," he presented the inner thoughts of the drug dealer. It was complicated because, like everyone else I knew, I still aspired to be those guys, even though they were also the force I blamed for destroying my family. Their cars had flash, their jewelry and watches gleamed, their clothes were top brand. They commanded respect and radiated a sense of status. We didn't have doctors and lawyers to look

---

* Nas, "The World Is Yours," *Illmatic* (New York: Columbia Records, 1994).

up to, or, more accurately, we didn't know about them. Our models of success were people like Jay-Z, guys who controlled their destiny, widened the parameters, and became something, whether mainstream society valued them or not.

My cousin Deuce was a successful drug dealer in Poplar Grove, and he colored a lot of my understanding of success. I just couldn't ignore how much power and control he wielded. I saw Deuce controlling the tester lines, his team, the flow in and out of the neighborhood. Since he held all the money, he held all the cards. Deuce was the center of the gravity.

Sadly, he met the inevitable fate of many dealers—killed at 22 by the same rules that propelled him to prominence. He was shot point blank multiple times while sitting in his car on Halloween night. I was 11 years old at the time of his murder, and it was a stain on my understanding of life in Baltimore. I was aware of the risks he took, but no one expected he'd get taken down so soon. He seemed larger than life, carrying a sense of power because he became someone in spite of his circumstances. There weren't many alternatives available, so he did what was necessary to create a life for himself. His death showed me that the life expectantcy of a young black man in the city of Baltimore was short, so I'd better make the most of the time I had.

After his death, Deuce became an even bigger deal, his reputation ballooning into legend status. If anything, in the warped world of the street, death cemented him in our collective consciousness. He was a fallen soldier.

⁣⁣

Years after I left school, I came across a line in *The Other Wes Moore* that felt like one of the truest statements I ever read: We are inevitably a product of other people's expectations of us.

On the bus ride home from Sudbrook, I would sit all the way up front by myself and not speak to anyone. One afternoon I was fuming, curdling myself up into a rage and kicking a metal emergency handle on the floor. *Swap!* I just kept kicking it, replaying some injustice from the school day.

"Little man," the bus driver said, looking through his giant rear view. "Quit that."

I kept at it. *Swap!*

"Yo, little man! Stop kicking!"

I ignored him, kicked harder, the clank against the floor echoing through the bus.

Swap!

"Little man!"

"Yo, mind your business," I snapped back.

"You making it my business!" he said. "Keep kicking and I'ma throw you off my bus."

"Throw me off the bus! I don't care," I said. Then, more to myself, "Life's not worth it anymore."

I stopped the kicking but my reaction must have alarmed him. When I stood up to get off at my stop, he put his hand out, blocking my exit. "Listen, man," he said, "I know you're going through something. Believe me, I've been there. But it'll get better."

The bus driver, whose name was Ben, started looking out for me, and he became something of a big brother. We'd talk MCs and mix tapes and lyrics. He had grown up without his father around, dropped out of school, had logged years as a drug dealer and stick-up kid in the Virginia projects, and was trying to turn his life around. There were so few people at Sudbrook who even seemed in my orbit that Ben stood out. And he expressed a genuine desire to get to know me. Some mornings he'd get us to school a little early and we'd sit there in the parking lot and talk, or I'd sit up front with him on the bus ride home and go over the day. Like Ms. Johnson, Ben was an island. He was an adult who took the time to look past the projection and see the real me in there, struggling to bust out.

Weekends at my grandparents' house were a respite. My grandparents lived in a row home in West Baltimore off the main strip. It wasn't much but it had personality and was given touches of care that made it a home. It had a bright yellow awning covering a cement porch that overlooked the small but well-kept yard, a silver chain-link fence encircling it. A small strip alongside the front steps was for my grandmother's seasonal flowers. During the day, we'd hear the toy-piano loop of the neighborhood ice cream truck, the barrage of loose laughter. The kids would have water gun fights on a patch of undeveloped land in the middle of the block that we called "The Park"—our own personal playground.

That home was an oasis, warm and welcoming; my grandfather was a blast to be around. He drove a sky blue and silver Thunderbird with tinted windows. He would pull up to their house with car windows down, blasting his favorite song:

Cotton candy, sweetie go, let me see the Tootsee Roll . . .

Then he'd get out and do the dance—shoulders spread, legs bending like noodles—and we'd all crack up laughing.

On the weekend, he'd host house parties and come to life playing host. He'd always invite his brother Jerry and a few of his buddies over to gamble on pool and dice. There was a pool table in the center of the basement, a huge stereo system, and a bar that was always stocked with vodka and Southern Comfort. The Al Green music would be turned all the way up, the cigarette smoke thick like fog. The drinks would be flowing and the shit-talking nonstop, its own battle being fought alongside the action.

"Mothafucka, you crazy! You can't fuck with me on this table!" my grandfather would say to his buddies as he sank ball after ball. "This is *my* house! You a fool thinking I'ma let your ass beat me in *my* house."

They'd laugh him off, knowing he was just getting started.

"Y'all black asses can't even beat my son. Shit, my grandson could beat y'all ass. Y'all definitely ain't fuckin' with me." He'd bust out this hearty laugh that rumbled up from his stomach. A full and inviting laugh.

My grandfather taught Jason and me how to shoot pool and play craps, and we got pretty good at it, especially against a bunch of older guys too drunk to see straight. Granddad would brag and hustle, betting we could beat his buddies. We'd win, and he'd let us keep the money, since it was all about bragging rights for him.

Late at night, a curtain would draw back on the city and the air would shift. After everyone went home, you could feel and hear it: ambulances whipping through the streets and police sirens washing over the night; screams of broken women and cold men; abrupt pops of gunfire. Sometimes I could shut it out. Other times, I couldn't. And then I'd think of my father.

Pop was present mostly as an absence during this time. There were still regular last-minute cancellations. Ready to go, I'd overhear my mother on the phone. "You gotta stop making promises to that boy you can't keep!" she would rail at him, as if she were talking to an empty line. In some ways, she was. "If you can't stick to your word, then you need to stop calling," she'd say. Eventually that's exactly what he did.

I still held out the irrational hope that he'd come around. I'd succumbed to nostalgia and inflated our moments together from my youth: walking to the corner store, having him treat me to Peanut Chews and penny candy. I even missed the scent of Jack Daniels on his breath and the menthol tobacco washed into his shirt. I didn't need Disney World; I would've been content with a trip to the community pool at Druid Hill Park.

It was like he had died on those street corners, but he would return, only to die over and over again. Each time he left, a part of me went with him. Fathers, even the most disappointing ones, automatically get that hero label early, and it takes a lot for them to shake it. In school, kids would trade off boasts about whose father was better, whose did what or could do what.

My father is a police officer and he gets to carry a gun.

My father is a fireman and he carried some lady out of a burning building.

Well, my father can build a whole car engine.

Well, my father is a doctor and he saved a guy's life.

Then the boasts would be followed by responses, takedowns:

Your father's not a fireman, he's too skinny to be a fireman.

He's so skinny he looks like a toothpick.

Well, your father's so old, he was friends with George Washington.

These snapping sessions would begin innocently, then quickly escalate into shoving matches if somebody's joke cut too deep. Fathers mattered that much because they were an extension of ourselves. I was sure that there'd be a change in fortune between me and Pop. Things would swing back, Pop would reenter my life, and I'd be ready.

〰〰〰〰〰〰〰〰〰〰〰〰〰〰〰〰〰〰〰〰〰〰〰〰〰〰〰〰〰〰〰〰〰

When I was 12, Pop was arrested for possession of drugs with intent to distribute and was sentenced to 6 years at Jessup Correctional Institute. He was an addict, not a dealer, but as far as the system was concerned, that distinction didn't matter. They didn't want to help people like him. They wanted to hide him.

Jessup Correctional is about half an hour south of Baltimore, in a rural area off the interstate. To me, it was an imposing industrial behemoth, red and white brick surrounded on all sides by nefarious barbed wire. The inside was all right angles, stone-faced men, and harsh lighting. My mother refused to visit Pop, so I went with my grandparents and Uncle Jason on the weekends, like a family activity. *Let's go see your father in prison.*

We'd park and walk across the dirt parking lot, dust kicking up. Then we'd go inside through the gated walkway into a silent little office with clean white walls, no sounds but the roar of the high-powered air conditioning. After writing down our names, the security guard would check our names against the list, then search us head to toe. We'd all empty our pockets, my grandmother would give over her bag—like airport security. A loud buzz, then another door, this time into a polished, shiny hallway that made all of our shoes squeak. We'd come into a giant cafeteria area with high ceilings, barred windows, and long white tables. Armed guards in starched blue lined the perimeter. Their eyes looked hollow, mean, and focused. Like they didn't see you but rather the threat you could pose.

A guard would escort us to a table and then walk over to the office. Through the glass, I would see them pick up a red phone. After about 10 minutes, there would be a buzzing, then a clanging, and a door on the other side would open up.

And then he would appear. It was always strange negotiating between the father in my head and the man who stood before me. There was Pop, wearing sweatpants and a T-shirt, worn sneakers or whatever my grandmother had sent him through the mail. He looked stockier, healthier—a positive effect of being off drugs on the inside. As time went on, he had started exercising, so he looked almost fit—as fit as I'd ever seen him.

Visiting him was painful. It was this heavy drag on my spirit, a physical thing I felt every time we pulled into that parking lot. My peers had a secure home with both parents, and I had to see my father in tight conditions in this horrible place, watched over by armed guards. There was even a no-touching rule. If I went to hug my father, the security guard would come over and separate us. Pop was right there—like through the passenger window—but I couldn't even touch his hand. There was a little photo setup in the corner for prisoners and their families, and sometimes we'd snap a family picture there.

The conversation was always strained. I was still young, and we didn't have a lot to talk about.

"How's school?"

"Fine."

Or, "How's your summer?"

"Fine."

Always, "How's your mom?"

"Good."

One time I mentioned how good he looked. He patted his stomach and looked surprised. "Really," he said, flashing that smile, a shadow of his old self.

"Well, I've been exercising. Pullups, pushups. The alcohol doesn't help."

"They let you drink in here?" I asked.

"Oh, hell no," he laughed. "They don't *let* us. It's pruno. Prison liquor. We gotta sneak it. We leave orange peels out, mix it with potatoes. It ferments like that."

"That works?"

"Gets the job done. Ask your science teacher about it." I saw him glance over at the clock on the wall.

My grandmother would step in and take my seat as I moved over. She and Pop would get down to what he cared about: his needs. They would go over how much commissary money he needed for things like cigarettes, where they were in the process of getting or keeping a lawyer, how his cases were going, and what could be done about his situation.

My sister Nicole, who was about 7 at the time, would visit with us sometimes. She would get hysterical every time we had to leave. It got to be too much—like a torture we were putting her through—so we had to stop bringing her. Once Nicole stopped visiting him, her mother stopped bringing her to my grandmother's house. Ten years would go by before I saw her again. Pieces of my family were being stripped away. Even locked up, my father was still doing damage.

A Letter

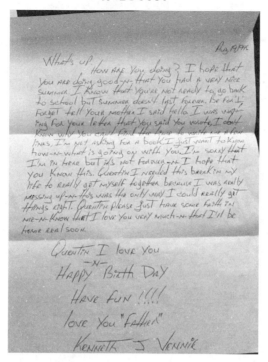

I was 13 and struggling to get through the day. Even basic things weighed on me so heavily that I felt I could barely breathe.

A few months after Nicole stopped visiting, things between my father and grandmother took a turn for the worse. I don't know the details, but he pushed my grandmother too far, and after years of picking up the pieces, she finally decided to let them remain where they were. She refused to visit for a while and took a break from sending him any money.

He would write me letters from prison, often explaining himself and saying how he needed prison to set some things right. He'd throw some blame my way for our strained relationship, writing things like, "I don't understand why you can't write me a simple letter." About what? I wouldn't even know where to begin.

CHAPTER
5

PROBLEM KID

THE SUMMER BEFORE I STARTED HIGH SCHOOL, my stress and anxiety began a full-frontal assault. Along with puberty and its hormonal onslaught, my emotional problems became physiological. The episodes first came as a rush in the middle of the night. A flush of heat would wash over my body, my heart rate would spike, and my chest would tighten as if my airways were closing. Dizziness would set in, then I'd begin to hyperventilate. It was terrifying, like my body was rebelling against me. I would get some ice water from the kitchen, lean against the sink, and try to get my bearings. But it wouldn't stop.

After the third or fourth episode, I ran into my mom's room and woke her up. I was starting high school in a few weeks, so she brushed it off.

"Maybe you had a bad dream, Quentin. You're just nervous about school. Go back to bed," she said. "Just try to relax." I did as she said—I *was* nervous about school—but something seemed dangerous. Like I was possessed. It felt like a fanged beast was trying to make room for itself inside my body.

The episodes kept happening, more frequent, more paralyzing. Like drowning in fresh air. The world was calm but my insides were at war. The more I wouldn't want them to happen, the more fiercely and frequently the attacks would come. First in bed at night, then when I woke up in the morning, then in all the spaces in between. I was afraid—and all the fear did was give the episodes more power.

After a few weeks, I convinced Ma it was serious. She agreed to take me to a doctor, who ran some tests and determined there was no physical trigger for my symptoms. He referred me to a psychiatrist, a tall guy in his mid-thirties with curly brown hair. Ma and I met him in a small office with smooth gray carpet and framed degrees and landscape paintings on the wall. There was the low buzz of the air conditioning and the distant sounds of kids playing in a park nearby. The doctor started low-key, like someone who was just curious about me.

"How do you like school?"

"School is cool."

"Yeah? You can be honest with me," he said.

"It's just school," I admitted. "For real, I'm not really into it."

"Why's that?" He had that unaffected demeanor that I would learn to expect from doctors. Poker-faced and noncommittal.

"I don't think they're teaching me anything important. When I apply for a job, they're not going to ask about the American Revolution," I said.

He smiled. "Perhaps not. And after school? Weekends? What do you do for fun?"

"Basketball. Hang out with my friends, go to the mall, movies. Listen to music."

"What kind of music do you like?"

I couldn't tell if he was interested or just pretending to be.

"Hip-hop," I said, unsure if he even knew what that was. "Rap. But I love all kinds of music."

He nodded a few times, wrote something down on the notepad resting on his lap. "Now, Quentin, I'm going to ask you something. Do you think you have a reason to be anxious?" The doctor had kind eyes, but there was something forced about him. Like he was reenacting something he'd read in a book. Like I was a subject he was studying.

"I'm not really nervous about anything. I'm not sure I know what being 'anxious' feels like," I said.

My mom, who had been trying not to interrupt, said, "Quentin, just tell him what's been going on."

"That's why we're here," he said.

"Okay." I was nervous, like talking about it would summon it into that room, wake up the resting beast. "Sometimes I just have trouble catching my breath, like I'm struggling to breathe. My chest gets tight, and then I'll get dizzy, just sitting still."

"Are you afraid when this happens?"

"Yeah, I'm scared." I looked over at my mother. "Every time it happens, it feels like I'm gonna die."

"So what do you do?"

"Try to calm myself down. Breathe deep, maybe get some cold water. If it doesn't go away, I'll just lay in the bed and cry. Pray that I live through it." My mother looked pained.

The psychiatrist asked questions about my home life, about my father, which I answered like a teenager, curt and vague. I didn't mention that Pop was in prison. "We don't have a good relationship," I said. I had grown tired of even thinking about my father and embarrassed about what his life said about mine. Like I was guilty by association.

"Well, from your symptoms, it sounds like you have anxiety and some depression," he said. "That's very common in people who don't have good relationships with both parents." His eyes drifted up to my mother, who kept her hand on my shoulder. "I'm going to recommend a course of Prozac," he said, writing on a small square pad. He tore off the sheet.

"Wait, wait, wait," my mother said, bursting alive. "I understand there are some things going on with him, but after talking to him for ten minutes you're just gonna say that he's got anxiety and depression and you want to medicate him?"

He tried to hand the prescription to my mother. "I think this will help him," he said.

But his arm just held there in that space; my mother didn't reach for the slip. "No," she said, sternly. "I don't think it will."

My mother had always had a deep suspicion of medicine, so I rarely took any growing up. Whenever I had a fever, Ma would take a raw white potato, cut it up in quarters, and wrap the pieces around my wrists and ankles. The potatoes would eventually warm up, and the fever would draw itself out. I wouldn't have believed that it worked if I hadn't seen it myself.

She had grown up around addiction, had a family history of it, so the idea of putting me on a drug just didn't sit right with her. Plus, she had worked as a care provider to children and adults with disabilities my entire life, so she knew the medical system's penchant to overprescribe.

The psychiatrist exhaled. *Ah, one of these.* "I understand," he said, leaning back in his chair. "And why do you feel that way?" He was polite, but the condescension was thick, floating there in the room among all of us. My mother's face changed.

"All y'all want to do is prescribe medication. Diagnose and prescribe, that's all you people do. You don't—"

"Ms. Butler—"

"—offer any real help."

"Ms. Butler. Your son would benefit from a course of this medication. Trust me. It's the best solution right now."

"Trust you? Well, that's not gonna happen. I'm sorry. Let's go, Quentin." From the door, she turned back to the doctor. "My son is not going to be a zombie," she said. "He's not going to be an experiment for y'all. If that's all you offer here, then we'll just figure it out on our own." That was that. We both walked out.

Ma was silent the whole ride home, annoyed, so I didn't speak. But I felt closer to her in that moment. There was an unspoken agreement between us; we didn't know what was next, but I took comfort in knowing I wouldn't be alone.

〰〰〰〰〰〰〰〰〰〰〰〰〰〰〰〰〰〰〰〰〰〰〰〰〰〰〰〰〰〰〰〰

That summer, Sudbrook invited some students to hear Dr. Ben Carson speak at nearby Towson University. For more than two decades, Dr. Carson was a hero in the eyes of Baltimore, black and white citizens alike. He was the first neurosurgeon to successfully separate conjoined twins; for him to have lived in Baltimore and done it here really shined a positive light on the city. He showed kids that anything was possible. He was the hope that Baltimore so desperately needed at that time, so to have the opportunity to see him speak live was a major deal.

When we filed off the bus onto that college campus—huge fresh lawns, giant buildings of faded brick—my eyes popped widely. I'd had virtually no exposure to that world, and what I had seen told me it wasn't for people like me. But Dr. Carson had grown up in poor neighborhoods with a single parent. When he was 8 years old, his mother moved him and his siblings from Detroit to the Boston projects, and he went on to become a world-class neurosurgeon. His speech gave me a lift at the perfect time, right when things were starting to break down. I got back on that bus with a sense of purpose, with proof that an exit was possible. I picked up his book soon after and read it cover to cover, lying on my bed at night after dinner. He'd seen and lived in the same world I had, known people like my family and neighbors:

A lot of winos and drunks flopped around the area, and we became so used to seeing broken glass, trashed lots, dilapidated buildings, and squad cars racing up the street that we soon *adjusted to our change of lifestyle. Within weeks this setting seemed perfectly normal and reasonable.**

Dr. Carson came from nothing and turned it into something—he was Jay-Z with an MD and a PhD. His story wasn't just an inspiration—I read it as a ladder. I could actually envision the steps for myself. Because addiction was rampant in my family, I had thoughts of becoming a doctor. Not only would I get myself out, but I could help my family with their problems. I had the adolescent desire to be a superhero, swoop in with my degrees and solve everything, save everyone.

My mother wanted me to go to a Catholic high school, but I convinced her to enroll me in the local magnet high school, Milford Mill Academy, which was predominantly black. My experience at Sudbrook had given me little hope that I'd succeed at another mostly white school. At Milford, I enrolled in the high school's health program.

It was already a challenging class with lots of medical terminology, which was like learning a new language. My teacher Mrs. Miller and I bumped heads from the start. As the only male in the class, I stood out, and she just didn't seem to have any experience with the testosterone and hormones raging inside a 14-year-old boy. Some of it was my showing off for the girls, but she just seemed dismissive and spiteful toward me. Mrs. Miller was black, and somehow that made her rejection especially hurtful and confusing. Why was she making things harder for me when she knew how hard it already was? At Milford, everything seemed to escalate and enlarge: My problems were expanding beyond the racial divide.

I needed help but instead found conflict, judgment, and more labeling. I would specifically ask Mrs. Miller for help, but she'd use those moments to expose me, to publicly embarrass me. She'd call on me to answer questions I felt she knew I couldn't answer. I was 14, so rather than making a fool out of myself, I'd make jokes about it.

* Ben Carson, with Cecil Murphey, *Gifted Hands: The Ben Carson Story*, Mass Market Paperback (New York: Zondervan, 1996): 22.

"Quentin, do you know the part of the brain responsible for complex sensory and neural functions?"

"Now Mrs. Miller, you know I don't know the answer to that," I said sarcastically. The girls laughed.

"That's rude, Quentin. And unnecessary. Why can't you just—just—?"

"Just what?"

Snickers. Giggles.

"Why don't you stop clowning for the girls, who don't like you anyway, and look at page 36 for the answer," she sneered. "If you can find it." She mumbled something under her breath.

I found the answer: *cerebrum*. I didn't want to sound stupid mispronouncing it, so I took my sweet time sounding it out. I said it drawn out and exaggerated—partly as a joke, partly to protect myself: "*SE—RA—BREEM*?" The kids laughed and I'd like to think it was with me, not at my expense.

We'd go back and forth until either she asked me to leave or I stormed out. After enough of those battles, she just got mean: *You have issues. You need to be on medication. There's something wrong with you.*

One day early into the year, I was in ninth grade geometry class, which was mostly upperclassmen. I had dressed up: cream-colored Chaps shirt, blue jeans, and gleaming white Nikes that I obsessively kept clean with a toothbrush, like my father had taught me. There was a *splat* and we all looked to the window; kids were reaching over from the class windows next door and throwing things into ours. Another smack at the window, and raised laughter. Milk cartons and soda bottles exploded at the window. The teacher had no control over his own students, much less the kids next door. "Just ignore it. Ignore them," he kept saying. "Follow along on page 22. Tanya, can you read for us?"

Kids started to lean in and throw things into the classroom through the open windows. I got up and moved my seat along with the rest of the row. As I was crossing the room, I heard, "Quentin, heads up!"

As I turned, a 20-ounce soda bottle splattered all over my shirt. A group of hulking dudes in the back busted out laughing. I got permission to leave and called my mother from the pay phone, asking her to bring me another shirt on her lunch break. Then I hung up and stared at the phone for a minute, and I caught my reflection in that sliver of silver. I remembered what my cousin Derrick said to me when he heard I was going to Milford: "If you have any problems, make sure you call me."

Derrick was a successful drug dealer who used to live close by and once controlled an entire block off Park Heights Avenue. I called him, and a few hours later he came by the school. Derrick was in his late twenties, tall and skinny with slouched shoulders. He never raised his voice and never needed to. Everything was very matter-of-fact, business—even when it wasn't. As I was telling him what happened and who did it, he was looking around, hawk eyes taking it all in. He just nodded quickly, like he had it all figured out.

"Yeah, yeah," he said, eyes darting around. "I hear you. Okay, cuz, tell you this. If it happens again, you call me again." He reached into his jacket and pulled out a pocketknife and a pair of garden shears. "I'll cut their motherfuckin' fingers off and then they won't be able to throw shit," he said, giving me a dap and a smile. "You straight?"

"Yeah, I'm straight," I said.

A few weeks later, I was talking with a girl in the hallway when a bulky senior picked me up off of my feet and slammed me against the lockers. I saw his friend sneak over, take the girl by the arm, and walk her around. I tried to wrestle free, but the dude was too strong. "Chill, lil' homie," he said. "You're just gonna make it harder on yourself." I gave up and just dangled there. While my feet were still in the air, I knew I'd be calling Derrick again: *You don't know who you're fucking with*, I thought. Later that day, Derrick tracked me down.

I pointed the guy out up against his locker, and Derrick smiled. "Shit, I know that big-head motherfucker. Come on, cuz." He dragged me over by my sleeve.

They gave each other daps and started to talk. I stood there, still pretty pissed and embarrassed and ready to see some action. I didn't necessarily want Derrick to cut the guy's fingers off—I wasn't built to see something like that—but I was anticipating some kind of vindication.

"Listen," Derrick said, wrapping his arm around me. "This is my little cousin. Don't fuck with him. I need you to *look out* for him. Have his back. You feel me?"

The guy looked at me, confused, and I saw the wheels spinning in his brain. He couldn't figure the connection from Derrick to me.

"I got you," he said. "All good. No problem."

"That's what I thought. Good looking out," Derrick said, and then he was gone.

In my grandmother's neighborhood, I was intimately familiar with the negative parts of drugs: I saw it in the dead faces on the street corners and in the evisceration of my father. But Derrick was the flip side. He had made his name and a living off of it. Derrick didn't have the skills that high school told me I needed, but he was doing better than most. The people who were successful around Poplar Grove and Park Heights didn't have college degrees; they had criminal records. I knew drug dealers who made in one week what my teachers made all year. My mother's older sister was the only person I knew with a college degree, and she didn't make nearly as much as those guys.

In just a few moments Derrick had pulled some jujitsu, turned the guy's aggression inside out and in my favor, transforming the bully into my protector. With a few words, Derrick not only erased that problem but solved any future problems. *Shit*, I thought, *that's power*.

CHAPTER

6

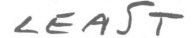

AT THE END OF NINTH GRADE, ALL OF THE students in my social studies class voted on unofficial awards. They had categories like Best Dressed, Smartest, Prettiest Girl, Worst Dressed, Best Couple. When we had the mock ceremony, I was called up to accept my one award: Least Likely to Succeed.

"Uh-uh," my mother said when I told her I wanted to transfer. It was after dinner and she was doing the dishes in the sink, weary from a double shift. "Not gonna happen."

"But I hate it there!"

"Not my problem, Quentin. You made your bed."

"What? What does that mean?"

She turned to me. "You made the decision to go to this school, you're going to live with it. You convinced me to let you go there. Now you ride it out."

"I'll just stop going then," I said.

She threw some silverware down in the sink and turned to me. "Oh, that's what you think?" she said. Her body clenched, her hands gripping the end of the counter. "I'm gonna pretend I didn't hear you just say that. I didn't raise no dropout, Quentin."

I had thought going to a black school would mean access to more people who looked and thought like me. In the early '90s, as hip-hop hit the suburbs, many suburban kids wanted to seem hard and street. The county kids at my high school started to imitate how they thought city kids were supposed to act, and the most popular of those kids were getting into trouble, smoking marijuana, and rolling dice in the bathroom. County students were suddenly causing problems just to fit in. It was a school of the phony leading the frauds, and it made me sick. All I saw were people pretending to be something they weren't.

The kids at my high school glamorized a life they knew nothing about—a life that actually terrified them. Derrick had exposed their phony front in about 5 seconds, which showed me how fragile those wannabe thugs really were. I had personal relationships with real drug dealers, criminals, and OGs from the old neighborhood. Some of them were members of my family. My cousin Deuce had been a generous guy, looking out for family and helping where he could. He'd give Uncle Jason and me a few bucks to go to the corner store and buy ourselves quarter waters, chips, and sunflower seeds. Those guys never glamorized that life. In fact, they would tell me to keep my grades up and stay in school, warn me *not* to look up to them.

My whole goal in high school was just to get out of it. *Head down, barrel through.* I never went to any school functions, sporting events, or pep rallies. I did keep writing. My closest friends were the only ones who knew how passionate I was about writing. For Black History Month, I wrote a poem for my 12th grade music class about Dr. Martin Luther King, Jr. I was asked to perform it for an after-school assembly, but I refused, pretending I couldn't take off from work. Truthfully, I had no desire to be a part of it. I was more concerned with making money than making grades. A fellow classmate read the poem on my behalf and received a standing ovation. Afterward, my music teacher, Mr. Percy, tried to convince me to write more poems for school projects, showcases, and assemblies, but I wasn't interested. I just wanted out of there.

Like a lot of kids who don't fit in, I held my breath and waited it out. I did just enough to get by, stayed under the radar, and decided to never reveal the real me. It became a game for me, portraying myself as less intelligent than I really was. I wanted to hide, avoid unwanted attention from my peers. I didn't want people asking me to help them or have teachers expecting more from me. I just wanted to do my 8–3, do enough work to pass, and get out. Nothing more.

I also had deep trust issues that throbbed in my veins and ran in my blood. I became a firm believer in hiding as protection, defense as offense: If people thought I wasn't smart enough to catch on to their game, then they would expose their true selves. Then I would have the upper hand. It wasn't until years later that I recognized the strain of that armor—it weighs you down and starts to choke you. It protects you so well that you suffocate under it.

Pop was still in prison, and we were visiting him less and less, but I still saw him all the time—in the faces of all the junkies in the old neighborhood, in the want and need that draped over them like ragged clothes. That was my *blood*, the line that I came from. Everything school had to offer and all its values became completely beside the point.

After school I would catch the bus out to Kendrick's Barber Shop, where I'd sweep hair for a few hours for some easy money. I didn't think I needed a diploma in order to make money, because I was *making* money. I knew virtually no one who graduated from college, and they all seemed to be living. When I floated these thoughts to my mother once over breakfast, I realized how little I knew. Though we never had money, Ma never complained about it. She talked about it so little, in fact, that I had no idea what it cost to live. Not until she broke it down for me.

"What do you bring home a week from sweeping hair?" she asked.

"One-fifty. Tax free," I smiled.

She wrote that down in a corner of the newspaper.

"Okay, what are your expenses?"

I showed her my new sneakers that I had bought with my own money.

"Okay, what were those, one-twenty?" She wrote that down. "What else?"

"I got my own line." That summer I had paid to have a second phone line installed in the house.

"Who feeds you?"

"You."

"Whose house is this?"

"Ours!"

"Yeah," she said with a slight smirk, "but who pays for it and everything in it?"

"You," I said.

"What if you break your arm? Who pays for the hospital?"

I lost momentum. I saw where she was going. "You."

While some of my classmates were preparing for college, others were taking their first steps into the criminal world. My mother knew what influences I faced at school and on weekends in the old neighborhood. She kept her feet planted where she was, hoping to latch me tight. But the temptations reared their heads.

On the first day of 10th grade art class, I met a kid named Roc; he was short and stocky with dark brown skin. When I first met him, he was growing his hair long to get cornrows, so he wore fitted caps to hide that awkward phase. We sat next to each other in the back of the class and, on that first day, while the teacher sorted out the seats, we got to talking.

"Where you from?" I asked.

"Park Heights."

"No shit. Me too!" I said. "Where you stay at?"

"The townhouses by the Windsor—"

"I know 'em—"

"—but I work at a car wash off of Wabash Ave," he said.

"You on the other side of the tracks? By the train station?"

"Yeah, past the train station going toward Garrison."

"Oh, so you at the car wash by the KFC."

"Yeah, man!"

Roc was like finding a rope that I could climb back to my past, or to a place where people knew the real me.

"I used to get in trouble for going across those tracks!" I said.

"Ha ha. I feel you, homie!"

We became fast friends. Roc was a huge jokester, so he commanded attention from cracking wise. He was usually lively and smiling, never taking anything too seriously. But he could switch in an instant. If he felt disrespected, he'd go into command mode and let people know he meant business.

A couple of weeks went by and we exchanged numbers, talked outside of school. Roc was already selling marijuana in school and had a Volvo, which was paid for. I was impressed that this 15-year-old kid was holding things down like that.

One day Roc came into art class disheveled and angry. I could tell something had gone down.

"What's up, G? You good?"

"Nah, I got into some shit," he said.

"What happened?"

"Some seniors took me off in the bathroom for some grass."

"Shit. What you going to do about it?"

He looked right into me, like there was no doubt in his mind. "I'm gonna see them."

"Yeah?"

"Shit, yeah. I got my pops and a couple of homeboys coming up here today before school ends." He opened up his backpack. "And I got this." A black 9mm glinted among his schoolbooks.

I tried to play it off, but the gun startled me, especially in the classroom. "Bro, you gotta do what you gotta do."

We started doing our work for class and he got called to the office, specifically told to bring all of his stuff. His father and uncle were coming to get him.

He looked at me and said, "My father don't know I have this. Can you hold it for me?"

I reached down and zipped opened my backpack. "Just put it in there," I said, sliding it over with my foot under the desks. I was out of my depth, but we were from the same place and lived by the same code. I implicitly trusted him.

I walked home from school with the 9 in my backpack and he called me later. He lived only 10 minutes away and came by to pick up the pistol.

It turned out Roc didn't even need it. He got the money and his product back without having to resort to it. I was relieved because I didn't really want to be part of something that went any further than that, especially when it didn't concern me. But from that day forward Roc and I formed a brotherhood, and we began to work some hustles.

I had moved on from the barbershop and was working after school in the men's department at Burlington Coat Factory. I used to pop the plastic sensors off the clothes with rubber bands and store the clothes in bags under some racks by the exit. Roc would swing by and grab them on his way out. We'd go to school the next day and sell everything: Phat Farm velour sweatsuits, cologne, watches, Ralph Lauren polo shirts, and V-neck sweaters. We made some serious money off that, way more than I ever made working for Burlington. It was an early lesson that the criminal life taught me, and what I was learning in school couldn't compete.

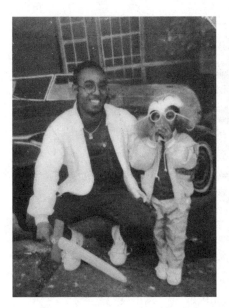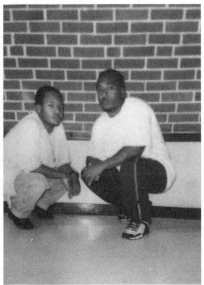

Meanwhile, Pop and I were going in opposite directions, like ships passing. After 4 years in prison he was transferred into a boot camp program, a more disciplined and structured part of Jessup. It was like a boarding school for convicts—and a stepping-stone toward release.

After completing that program, he was released into a halfway house in West Baltimore where former addicts and convicts received assistance and professional training. The goal was to reintroduce them into the world. It turned out I was something my pop tried to reintroduce himself to—and I just wasn't interested. By the time he was getting back on track and wanted a relationship with me, I was 15 and naturally on to other things.

The halfway house was a three-story building in a rundown part of the city, almost like a group home for adults. I always went with my grandmother and Jason and sometimes my aunt Nikki. We'd give our name to one of the staff on the first floor and he'd yell up, "Kenny, you have visitors!"

That house was always dark in the daytime, with a pallor that covered everything. Dust kicked up in the window light. The walls were a faded burgundy, the furniture holed-out donations from Goodwill. The paint was chipped and peeling, and the steps creaked like they just wanted to collapse. It was just an exhausted place, with no signs of life. Nothing about it felt like a place of resurrection.

All the people we saw looked like they belonged there. They carried it on their faces and it hung on their bodies—addiction, poverty, loss, pain. Pop was really trying to make the transition and stood out as one of the guys who showed promise.

We hung out in the downstairs living room, which served as the waiting area. He walked down the steps, gave everyone a hug, and sat down in the living room. I didn't really like to sit down there so I just stood up, usually leaning against a wall.

On my first visit he looked healthier, filled-out, in better spirits—though he just hated being there.

"So how is everything?" my grandmother asked.

"It's all right," he said, trying to straighten up magazines on the coffee table before giving up. "Dirty as shit in here." Aside from his few years as an active addict, he had always been a neat person. He was the one who taught me how to clean my sneakers with a toothbrush when I was 6 years old.

"What you been up to?" Jason asked.

"Not much. I don't have a phone, so it's not like I can talk to anybody. I can't go nowhere. But I'm making it," he added. "It's better than where I was, you know?" It was like he needed to show gratitude, stay on karma's good side.

As for our relationship, in my mind he had blown it. I needed him when I was 10, and he wasn't there. Now I was 15, had my confidence, my own circle of friends, and my own interests. It was good he was getting his life together but why should I sacrifice? I had already lost years of time and effort on him, and now he's coming around? I was in high school, had a girlfriend, making money boosting clothes, having sex for the first time. I just didn't have the energy to care about his side of things.

Plus every visit was about him wanting something, his needs, about "when am I gonna get out of here?"

Usually at the end of the visit, he'd take me aside and out of my grandmother's earshot. "Damn, nice kicks, Q," he said once. I was wearing Nike Air Force 1 high tops with the ankle strap.

"Thanks. Just got them."

"Oh yeah, you got a job now?"

"Yeah, working over at Burlington four days a week."

"Very cool. Good."

There was a silent pause, hovering over us. Then he said, "I need to get a pack of cigarettes. You got a couple dollars on you? I'll make sure I get it back to you."

I hated seeing him without, and I think he knew that; I'd always give him what he asked for. But it was like he saw me working as a way for him to get money, which hurt. Even his own son was not spared from this habit.

My father would often seem to guilt people into giving him things. He hadn't lost that skill in prison, and I was one of the main people he used it on—it was as if I was punished for visiting him. It was one of the reasons I stopped going there.

I got tired of hearing about how prison had made him a better person and he loved me and that he was hoping we could get a relationship restarted. Everything out of his mouth just felt like an excuse that he used to justify his mistakes and to explain away why he hadn't contributed anything positive to my life. He didn't know how badly I was hurting on the inside, and I didn't feel the need to tell him because there was nothing he could do. He didn't even know me. How could he?

I started spending more time at my aunt's house, my mother's older sister, hanging out with my older cousin Xavier and his friends, who introduced me to marijuana. One time his friends were hanging out in the backyard and as I came out, they were all laughing at something I'd missed. One of them, wearing sunglasses in the overcast day, turned to me and said, "Have you ever smoked a fug?"—a cigarette.

"Nah, I never tried that."

"But you get high, yeah?"

"No doubt," I lied.

"You smoke a fug afterwards cause it'll boost your high."

"Cool, cool," I said.

Once they thought I got high, they invited me to join them. The first time it was awkward, then it was terrifying. I was paranoid, afraid I was going to get caught, worried my aunt was going to come home and smell it on me. They spent half the time laughing at me and the other half trying to calm me down.

"Yo Q, chill out. You acting weird and people are gonna know."

My heart was sprinting and I felt like I was going to die. "I can't breathe," I kept saying. "I can't breathe." I can't imagine why I tried it again, but I did. And again.

After a few more times, the paranoia subsided and I was able to relax. Once that pleasant high kicked in, I was into it. It calmed me down and wiped away my worries: my father, school, grades, everything. I'd kill hours eating Doritos and laughing incessantly. Then I got tired and went to sleep. It was my first taste of chemical escape and I loved it, a refuge out of myself. I started staying out late, going with Jason into clubs in the city to see our friend Reddz DJ, and getting drunk. The pull of that life, that mental escape, was magnetic.

In the spring of 11th grade, I was called into my guidance counselor's office. She worked out of a tight, overstuffed room with nowhere to sit. She had a few pictures of her family on her desk. On the green walls hung her college degrees, generic framed landscape posters, and laminated motivational slogans, peeling away.

"Quentin," she said, as she searched her desk for my file, "have you done any thinking about college?"

"Well—"

"Because you know the opportunities for you will open up, and though your grades are not up to par, there's still time in the year. So if you—"

"I've been thinking that—"

"I've seen enough kids come into that door who had given up way too early on themselves," she said. "And it just doesn't make sense to do that. I mean to your future self, you understand?" She was an older black woman with glasses, a little overweight, with moles on her face. She looked up at me through her glasses, as if for the first time. She must've noticed something on my face because her expression changed. She went off script.

"Everything okay with you?" she asked.

"I guess."

"So," she said, sipping her coffee, "college. What are your thoughts?"

I knew what I was supposed to say, but I couldn't even fake it. "Nah," I said, "I'm not really interested in going to college at all. But my mother wants me to, so I don't know. I still might."

"Well, I'm just putting you on alert," she said, pushing the papers to the side. "At this rate, you may not graduate."

For whatever reason, that was all it took. It wasn't much of a motivational speech, but the threat of disappointing my mother—who had done so much for me—was enough. The one promise I made to her was that I would graduate from high school. That mattered to her. So it mattered to me.

My change in the classroom was instantaneous. All I did was apply myself; the work was easy. School had never been difficult. I still had that "me against the world" mentality, but the work itself was cake. I got my diploma, and even completed one semester of college, but after that, I dropped out. I gave up on myself, figured I wasn't going to make it out, so I cut my losses. The years of being told that I wasn't good enough had weighed me down. The degradation had taken its toll. I felt like a failure.

PART II

COBRA
POSE

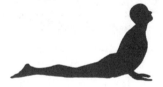

The nursing child will play by the hole of the
cobra, And the weaned child will put his hand
on the viper's den.

ISAIAH 11:8

THIS POSE IS A BACKBEND resembling a serpent with its hood raised. It strengthens the spine. It also expands the openness of the chest, stretching the shoulders broadly and the abdomen simultaneously.

CHAPTER
7

MOE

"ALL RIGHT, YO. BE STRAIGHT WITH ME, Q."

"What's up, Roc?" I said. "When you know me not to be straight?"

"Do you just need money? Or do you want to get put on?"

He was hesitant, questioning my motives, but I had already thought this through. I knew the answer.

Neither my heart nor my mind had been into college. High school graduation was a period, a definitive end; I had trudged and trekked and reached the summit. A huge relief flowed through me that day and there was just nothing left in the tank. I had made good on my promise to Ma and that was that. I enrolled in college only because I thought it would please her—she had to drop out when she got pregnant with me—but even my duty to my mother couldn't get me back in the classroom. All those years of school had left me a husk of myself. Now, I had to build myself back up on my own.

Virtually no one I knew even tried college, which devalued it in my eyes: I didn't feel like I needed it to be an adult. I was living in an apartment with my girlfriend Christina in Owings Mills, a quiet suburb of Baltimore. I had a full-time job, first as a valet and detailer at a car dealership, where she also worked, and then doing collections for a financial company. I had built a humble but sustainable life on my own when the bottom dropped out from under me.

I was 19 going on 20 when I lost my job; right on the heels of that, Christina lost hers. One of us out of work was a problem; both was an emergency. We ran smack into a wall and needed money fast. Moving back in with my mother was out of the question; I had far too much pride for that kind of lurch backward. Back when I was still living at home, Ma and I had a big blowout when I asked if Christina could live with us. "Well, screw it, then," I said. "Then I won't stay here either. We'll just both find somewhere to go." And that's what we did. I had a chip on my shoulder, and I felt like I had to prove myself as an independent man.

"Naw, I need a shot—an opportunity," I told Roc on the phone that day. "I need you to put me on with something."

In the 2 years since high school, Roc and I had hung out regularly, so I knew he'd been making good money dealing. Roc knew me as a hustler— always carving out ways to make money—but he initially had trouble viewing me as the dealer type.

"All right," he said. "All right. That's what I needed to hear." His tone changed, from friendly to business, like flipping a switch. "No more talking on the phone. I'll come by your crib and we'll run through it."

A few days after our phone call, he came by my apartment when Christina was out at the store. Roc had come into his own, wearing his newfound power like tailored clothes. He was still the same funny guy—quick to bust someone up with a joke—but it was more precarious. There was a low menace now, a cautiousness that betrayed his livelihood. Getting deeper into the streets can turn the most lighthearted person into a monster.

It was a transformation with which I'd soon become intimately familiar.

In my living room, Roc was peeking out the drapes, as though there was something to see. "So I gotta ask, Q," he said, "why now?" He and I already had a tight bond, but I think the interrogation came from his curiosity. I walked him through the situation.

"If I don't find something quick," I said, "I'm fucked. For real. We'll have no place to stay. And hell no I ain't going back to my mom's house."

"I hear you," he said, with a loose laugh. He was walking around the room, peering at different photographs on the walls. "Well, good thing I'm already out here in the Milli"—that's what we called Owings Mills—"so I'll set you up with my people. The first thing you need to do is buy a burnout phone, prepaid. Nothing that can be traced."

"Right," I said.

"Do that today. Like right after I leave."

"Okay."

"And you need a nickname." He sat down across from me on the easy chair. He leaned forward and started tapping his fingers on the glass table. "You can't have any of these fiends knowing your government, nothing about you. Don't tell them you live around here—ever. And if you get caught up in trying to reason with them, they'll see you as weak. Start to take advantage of you. Plus—"

"Roc," I said, "I appreciate all this, for real. But I don't need Junkie 101. I dealt with my father for like ten years. I got a PhD in that shit."

"True, true," he laughed. "All right then, you good." He stood up and gave me a dap. "Go get the phone and meet me back here in like two hours."

When he came back, Christina and I were watching TV on the couch. "Let's go for a ride," he said, holding open the front door. "I'ma introduce you to a few people." Christina didn't even look up when we left. I didn't tell her where we were going and she didn't ask.

Roc had sold the Volvo he'd owned in high school and was now driving a souped-up Chevy Tahoe, fresh green paint job and chrome rims. We peeled down the street, 50 Cent blaring on his new stereo. "I gotta drop off some packages, so you gonna just ride with me and meet these people."

"They live here?"

"Shit, man. They all live out here. The Milli is a gold mine, son," Roc said. "So much money out here and it's untouched. An untapped market." Roc was exploiting a bulging customer base; the residents in this part of town were mostly professionals with disposable income. These weren't your textbook junkies; a lot of them were low-key drug users. But they were using enough that Roc actually needed to bring someone else in to manage the flow.

As 50's "Many Men" was bumping in his car, bleeding through the sub-woofer in the back, Roc barely looked at the road. He reached over and turned down the radio.

"So, what're you thinking for your name?"

"How about Moe?" I said, staring at the suburban houses flying by. Same after same.

"Mo? Like M-O? Like Mo' Money?"

"Naw. M-O-E," I said.

"Ah, Moe. Moe," he said to himself, seeing if he liked the sound. "That works. So my boy Black is handling the crack, so I'm going to make you the dope connect."

"Sounds good," I said. "I appreciate it."

"You're my man, Q," he said, flipping serious again. "I always got you."

We drove up to a big white house on a tucked-away suburban street, a neglected single-family home that was barely standing. A row of skinny addicts was shuffling in and out the door, a pack of them sitting around the porch. Black shutters covered the windows and choked-out grass spotted the front yard. A layer of dirt covered everything like a coat of paint: the beat-up cars, the toys scattered in the yard, the bikes laying like corpses on the porch. Beer cans were lined underneath the porch railing all the way up the wooden steps.

"Wait here," Roc said, stepping out of the car. Some of the porch hangers chatted with him on his way in. Five minutes later, he came back out with a frail white woman trailing behind him, as if on a string. I stepped out to meet her. She had long grisly hair and could've passed for 50-something, though she couldn't have been older than 30.

"Jenny," Roc said. "This is Moe. Your new connect. He'll be taking care of you from now on."

It was strange being introduced as someone else, someone I'd just invented on the way over there. Jenny's eyes were empty saucers.

"Jenny!" Roc said sharply. She reached out a veiny hand, and I quickly shook it, unnerved by her ghostly touch. As I gave her the number to my burnout phone, she took a pen from Roc and wrote it on the back of her hand.

"Jenny's good people," Roc said, as though she wasn't there. Her eyes were wandering over to his car, the sky, across the street to a better version of her house. "And she knows everyone in the Milli. So you're set."

I knew if this girl was going to be my main connection—that my livelihood was tied to her—I needed to give her an incentive. I told her that for every hundred dollars she helped me move, I'd give her a free hit. She nodded and wandered back into the house. Roc and I got into the car and repeated this a few more times, him introducing me as Moe, me giving out my phone number. As simple as that, I was employed again.

I had grown up in the orbit of drug dealers and street deals, so that opportunity was always hovering there for me. But I held out because I was dead set against ever standing on the corner. I'd spent time with those guys, saw what kind of attention they drew, what their day was like, how exposed they were.

When I was 11, I was with Jason and some friends outside the Chinese carryout near my grandmother's house. We were eating beef and broccoli out of oyster pails, laughing about something, when this pack of older kids ran up on us. "Stick-up boys!" someone yelled out. Then *pap, pap, pap,* a quick run of shots that sounded like firecrackers on the pavement.

We all scattered down the alley and up the street, like pigeons bursting outwards. Jason and I ran back toward my grandma's until our breaths sputtered out. The memory clenched at me in my gut and kept my eyes wide open. Just the fact that I had been standing there that day made me a target. Even broke and desperate, that was no life for me. But now, the whole thing was a basic equation. I had been going to work every day, 40 hours a week, making $10 an hour, $800 every 2 weeks before taxes. Now I'd be making around $800 for a couple hours of making calls and hanging around the local gardening store, dropping bags behind mailboxes and inside newsletter vendors, and collecting money. It was a no-brainer.

When I called Roc, I didn't think I would be in the game long term. Virtually no one plans on going into the drug trade. Your options start to run out and then you fall into it, through a mix of desperation and opportunity. Like so many others who had grown up in similar circumstances, I had come up against the impenetrable. I just felt I had no other options. Instead of hitting the pavement and wasting time filling out job applications and going on interviews, I had a trusted friend willing to rope me in to a good situation for better money.

Roc provided me with consignment, like a loan on product. He wanted a specified amount of money off each package of heroin, which was pre-bagged; I had a little wiggle room regarding price, but my territory was prescribed. There was a convenience to working close to home, but the downside was the lack of separation: I was right on top of my customers. Plus, dealers did real time in the county—nothing was thrown out or suspended. There were no slaps on the wrist, or cases backlogged like at the central booking downtown. If you got caught with drugs in Baltimore County, you were going to jail.

It was easy to get adjusted to life as a dealer. I set my hours and just waited at home for my phone to ring. All my clients knew my time cap: I'd answer it between 8 a.m. and 8 p.m. Jenny was my main source, so most of my deals came through her. I didn't have to worry about too many people knowing me or having face-to-faces with junkies I didn't want to know. I embraced being Moe, I loved it—the mystery, the protection. Plus, the money was undeniable. I went from making about $400 a week to making that in less than 2 days. I paid my rent up for the next 4 months, paid Christina's car payment up for 6 months, and then splurged on a few things like expensive dinners and Iceberg outfits.

But as business rapidly expanded, a quiet voice was getting too loud to ignore. I was growing uncomfortable with the risk I was taking out in the county. Every pass off, every ride home, I had the distinct feeling of being tailed or watched. Every Crown Vic that passed, every Chevy Malibu at a stoplight—they were all converging on me. Whether it was in my head or not, the money just wasn't enough to cover the risk.

The paranoia reached full tilt one afternoon, about 6 months into my time under Roc. A few blocks from my apartment was an Exxon, which was next to a Frank's Nursery & Crafts store, a regular spot where I met customers. My routine was to park my car, a gold Nissan Altima, in the gas station by the vacuum and air pumps. Then I'd walk over to Frank's parking lot to conduct my business.

That day I pulled into the Exxon with nearly $1,000 worth of heroin hidden inside the gear shaft of my car. As I drove up, I saw a black Crown Vic in my regular spot, the windows tinted and the car running. Something felt off about the car in that spot and an ominous feeling crept slowly up my neck. I parked at a pump, took $5 in gas, and went inside to pay, trying to get a closer look at the driver of the car or see if someone inside could be pinned as its driver. No one was inside the gas station.

My customer kept ringing my phone. "I'm close," I said when I picked up. "Five minutes." I wanted to make sure I wasn't being watched.

Still on the phone, I got back in my car and told my customer, a scraggly white guy, to walk inside the nursery and go into the soil aisle, figuring his look wouldn't draw undue stares there. "I'll meet you," I said, "but don't approach me."

I pulled out of the gas station going away from Frank's, U-turned in the next lot, and tried to see if the Crown Vic followed me. It didn't, and when I rode by the gas station again, the car was gone. I pulled into Frank's and backed into the space right next to the customer's car so that our drivers' sides were adjacent. I took the heroin from the gear shaft, put it in a small black plastic bag, tied it, and tossed it underneath his car. I walked into Frank's and spotted my guy, then I rang his cell and gave him instructions: leave the money under a bag of soil on the second shelf. Walk out to your car, but stay on the phone.

He left the money, and I swooped in right behind him. I snuck to another aisle to quickly count it, and then told him where his product was before hanging up. Through the store window I watched him pull off, then I bought a small plant and walked out. As I was getting into my car, the Crown Vic passed right in front of Frank's and kept going. I was lucky, but I knew I likely dodged a bullet.

"Bro, shit is getting too hot for me," I told Roc on more than one occasion. "I'm not sure how much longer I can do this."

Because of our relationship, Roc was cool with it. He had put me on as more like a favor; he wasn't going to try to stop me if I wanted out. However, this was not normal for the drug trade. Once someone is brought into the operation, like with any illegal enterprise, it's not smart to just let them go. But I was one of the few people Roc actually trusted; he knew I would take a bullet for him.

After a few conversations like this, we agreed that it would be best that I step away. And with that, I felt like my short stint in the street life was done.

But a couple of weeks later, I started talking with an older guy named Laurence who lived in my great-grandmother's neighborhood. He was in his mid-thirties, half Hispanic, half black, light-skinned with curly hair. He had a deep, James Earl Jones baritone and a large presence, though he wasn't much taller than me. He just had that command of space. He knew Uncle Jason and me already, so there was a built-in relationship. Laurence dealt in heroin, just like Roc, but his operation wasn't in the suburbs: He operated in the city and offered me an opportunity too good to pass up.

"I'ma put you on for real," he told me. "Take it to the next level. Partners, son. Fifty-fifty." Laurence recruited me with the hard sell, offering me an even split and incentives. Unlike being with Roc, where there were different people handling different parts of the business, Laurence and I would be controlling the entire operation.

"Shit, for real?" I asked.

"You know it, Q. No man can make it alone," he said solemnly. He was good to his word.

All my jobs in the straight world had been musty dead ends. With Roc, and then with Laurence, I felt the openness of reaching my potential, and I thrived. Laurence only had city customers and he actually liked that I lived in the county, which gave our business a safe haven and a cover. No one would ever expect what we were doing on our family block crowded with Big Wheels, minivans, and nine-to-fivers.

"I'm going to show you everything you need to know," Laurence told me, treating me more like an associate than an employee. "How to mix the product, what to mix it with, what number to put it on"—how much to cut the heroin's potency—"everything you need to know about the game. And I'm going to make sure you make a lot of money."

I mixed and bagged the product, met the connects, and initially didn't have to sell anything to anyone. Laurence and I made drops to other dealers and collected the money. It was less time with customers and less risk.

Heroin is either snorted or injected through a hypodermic needle. I sold it in powder form, not in its raw state. What I sold was called scramble, heroin cut with other things like bonita and quinine, which were essentially baby laxatives. We'd throw things like morphine into the mix in order to increase and extend the high. Part of the game is knowing how much you can stretch it out—maximize it—without customers feeling like they're getting ripped off or causing an overdose. No dealer wants an overdose; it's not because of compassion, it's because of money. Once the street traced it back to your product, no one would buy it. An overdose is a huge liability to the business.

Laurence had actually been looking for a way out and was hunting for someone he could hand his business over to in due time. So he was grooming me, to an extent. But first, he had to make sure I knew the game in and out.

That first week, Laurence gave me a copy of Sun Tzu's *The Art of War*.

"What's this?" I asked.

"A book."

"No shit," I said. "What's it for?"

"Read it. Cover to cover." He tapped his meaty hand on it. "Every principle in that book will teach you about the drug trade."

I stared at the author's foreign-sounding name and the title. "A book about war?"

"Fuck yeah," he said.

Laurence just had a magnetic pull that made you want to buy in. I went home that night and started plowing through *The Art of War*.

I was astounded. Sun Tzu lived in 500 BC, and had never slung heroin to my knowledge, but his words just penetrated right into the game. I found myself underlining things on just about every page.

All warfare is based on deception.
Supreme excellence consists in breaking the enemy's
resistance without fighting.
He will win who knows when to fight and when not to fight.

The Art of War addressed the precarious balance that fosters success, the equal dangers of recklessness and cowardice—two sides of the same coin. He warned against the "delicacy of honor, which is sensitive to shame; and a hasty temper," all of which were fatal flaws on the street. I knew more than a few people who had been taken down or taken out because of them.

The book transcended dealing. It seeped into me on another level: my internal struggle, my strategy for survival, my need to hide my true self as a form of power.

At first then, exhibit the coyness of a maiden, until the enemy gives
you an opening; afterward emulate the rapidity of a running hare,
and it will be too late for the enemy to oppose you.
O divine art of subtlety and secrecy! Through you we
learn to be invisible, through you inaudible, and hence
we can hold the enemy's fate in our hands.

The book brilliantly laid out the psychology behind winning any battle. It meshed with my mentality, how I'd viewed my dynamic with the world since I was 10 years old. It was all a battle, whether external or internal. Sun Tzu focused on how to take responsibility, how to lead, when to change your view and shift your perception, how to read others, how to approach things strategically. I ate it up.

On Saturdays, Laurence and I would hit up the Patapsco Flea Market to buy the gel casings that we used to transport and distribute the product.

We'd buy five bags of 500 caps each and be set for the week. In Baltimore, the heroin was generally low-grade and brown, but Laurence knew people up in New York City who could get better-quality product. The heroin up there was a much purer charcoal gray.

One Friday night, we drove the 4 hours up I-95 to Spanish Harlem, spent the night in a roach motel, and hit up a string of bodegas and convenience stores—all fronts for drug operations. We came through with stacks of money and bought our heroin, morphine, and bonita and quinine in bulk. Eventually we started meeting our Harlem connect on the outskirts of New York City, then Newark and Philadelphia. From those trips, our operation expanded quickly. Laurence and I also evolved into other drugs, like crack cocaine and marijuana, as well as other parts of the country, mostly down south, where drug prices are way cheaper and we could resell in Baltimore with a huge markup.

Laurence's cousin in Tennessee kept telling him how cheap the product was down there. It's well known in the drug world that product is cheaper in the South, just like everything else. Having someone connected in its underworld, we took advantage. We traveled down to this nothing town outside Memphis and met up with our connect: a perpetually hyper guy who looked like Lil' Flip, light-skinned with cornrows, gold fronts, and tattoos. He was always drinking lean, a sedative, which is promethazine and codeine cough syrup mixed with Sprite and Jolly Ranchers. Flip would walk around sipping the purple juice out of a baby bottle. The first time I saw him doing it, I leaned forward from the back of the car and asked, "Yo, why you drinking out of a baby bottle?"

He smacked his lips. Then he looked through the rearview with a sly smile. "You gotta sip slow, baby."

Initially I had conflicted feelings about being a dealer. I'd think, *This person is someone's father or someone's mother. I'm taking food out of a kid's mouth.* Laurence was astute, practically a mind reader. He caught on to these rumblings in my conscience. As a veteran, he could smell doubt and knew how to shut it down. When he sensed me straying, he'd return to the same tactic. "You gotta stop looking at them as people," he'd say to me. "They're not people anymore, Q. They're not people."

Laurence's words started to percolate. My natural sympathy and compassion got muffled, then drowned out. If customers didn't get it from me, I rationalized, they were just going to get it from somebody else. It didn't start with me and I certainly couldn't end it. Why not get as much as I could for me and mine? The trick, Laurence taught me, was to become a wall—no weak spots, no openings.

One of my regular customers was Jojo, a scrawny guy who drove a raggedy Ford pickup and often bought $500 or $600 worth of heroin at a time. Once he didn't have all the money and asked for a loan on it. "I'll bring the extra hundred when I buy again," he said.

"Sure, no problem," I said. It was a slippery slope, but I trusted him, saw him regularly, and knew he was good for it. He came back with the extra hundred the next time, but then a month later he wanted the same deal. I did it again, but this time he vanished. Months passed.

Then, out of the blue, Jojo called Laurence to buy $500 worth of product, not knowing he and I were partners. Laurence called me up immediately. "I think this is your man that beat you for that hundred," he said. "What are you trying to do about it?"

"No shit," I said. "When you meeting him?"

"A couple hours."

"All right," I said. "I'ma bring you something and then we'll get his ass." I blended up some coffee grounds and flour, put it in gel caps, and packed it in a small plastic bag. Then I grabbed my baseball bat and drove out to meet Laurence at a parking lot we used. I passed over the bags. "You go ahead and serve him," I said. "Get the money and I'ma be in the bushes by the gate."

Jojo showed up, made his transaction, and headed back to his truck.

As he put his hand on the door handle, I ran up and swung the bat at the base of his neck. He fell forward, smacking into the side of his truck—*thwack*—and rolled onto his back. I looked straight at him, the whites of our eyes meeting in the dark, and said nothing. He covered his face, begged me not to hit him again. I just stood there, held it for a moment so he saw my face clear. I got back in my car and went home, tossing the bat back in my closet. It wasn't about the money. It was the fact that he thought he could get over on me—that message travels, and in our business, your reputation is your livelihood. Violence was never really my style, but everyone had to prove themselves on the streets. It is also bad for business, a liability that only brings unwanted attention. Jojo had left me no choice but to play enforcer.

Going at Jojo like that was something of a turning point. I felt a change, found reserves of anger and coldness I didn't know I had. Once you draw from that well, you see how deep it actually is. It also becomes automatic, almost natural. Laurence's voice cycled in my head: *You gotta stop looking at them as people. They're not people anymore.*

I was trained to be heartless, like a soldier who learns to become another self in battle. You forget about the life you had and are only focused on surviving. But while soldiers fight to return to their old lives, we were fighting to never go back to ours. When faced with the possibility of losing credibility, you had to become someone else. You had to protect who you were ultimately trying to become.

My disdain for the customers came from a deeper place. I don't know how conscious of it I was, but in hindsight I can see how I was feeding off the anger I'd felt all those years toward my father. I was projecting my frustration onto them, almost imagining them to be my father, knowing that there was a child on the other side of this transaction who was being let down. I was like a vigilante, punishing the parent on behalf of the child. At the same time, I was proving myself to myself, erasing that timid 10-year-old waiting for his father to pick him up, crying, and leaving himself open to getting let down again. The whole process turned me ugly: I had to become something of a monster.

‖‖

One summer, the heroin well had dried up. It's a common occurrence in the streets—a drought on product. There could've been a huge drug bust from one of the major distributors, or things could've been too risky to collect on a drug order. There's a hierarchy in the drug trade, just like in corporate America. So if our connect was unable to reach his connect, everything shut down: There was no product to sell.

A great deal of the violence in the trade grows out of these periods of desperation. A rival dealer who has a way to get product when you can't starts to take your clientele, and wars happen. Addicts aren't loyal to anyone or anything but their habit. Instead of me and Laurence shooting our way out of the problem, we opted to shift to marijuana, which Flip—down in Tennessee—could sell us in bulk.

Laurence and I were staying at a chain hotel on the outskirts of Memphis, part of the nameless stretch of franchises on the interstate. Flip picked us up and drove us the 30 minutes into the city, to an apartment complex. He gave us a key to one of the apartments. "Just chill in there," he said. "I'll be back with my connect."

The apartment was completely empty: no furniture, no television, no air conditioning. Laurence and I waited there, hot and bored. Time rolled out slow, and we started to get nervous. Flip knew how much cash we were carrying; he could've been planning on robbing us, killing us, or both. We sat on the floor, up against the white walls, and just waited. Sweating. After about 2 hours, a knock on the door pierced the quiet. The noise startled even Laurence, who didn't get startled at anything.

"C'mon out," Flip said casually. Laurence and I followed Flip out front. He led us to a black car with tinted windows, a faceless man behind the wheel who didn't turn around, didn't even move. The trunk popped open, revealing 10 lawn-sized trash bags. "Take one," Flip said. Laurence grabbed one of the black bags and we walked back into the empty apartment. We dumped the bag out, and 30 pounds of marijuana tumbled onto the hardwood floor, pyramiding into a big pile.

We gave Flip the money, he signaled the car through the window, and the faceless driver peeled off. We grabbed our half of what was on the floor and threw it back in the bag, then Flip took us to a housing project deep in the hood to get our weed compressed and repackaged to ship back home. Flip knew guys who would use vacuum pack machines to suck all the air out so that it wouldn't smell and the bag wouldn't burst during transport.

It was a rundown set of buildings, their faded blue and white paints peeling. Young kids played on the sidewalk while smoldering dudes huddled outside their cars, blasting music in clouds of pungent smoke. We walked up four flights of stairs inside one of the brick buildings.

When we walked into the apartment, everyone stopped and looked at us. Three Jamaican guys with heavy accents were on the black leather couch playing PlayStation on a big-screen TV. On the coffee table was a revolver and two 9mm semiautomatics, casually lying next to a giant silver bowl filled with marijuana. Each dude was smoking his own thick blunt and passing it in a circle, working a three-man rotation. Machetes were propped up on the walls like pieces of art, and a shotgun was leaning behind the front door.

I'd built some street armor in my time, but I was shaking in my sneakers. We were on these guys' turf, carrying 15 pounds of marijuana and hefty rolls of cash. My heart racketed around as I struggled to hide all signs of fear. My first instinct was that I was going to be killed. I'd heard of way too many people being set up and killed during drug deals. That scene was like out of a movie, right before someone gets robbed and shot. Except it was real.

I tried to catch Laurence's eye, wondering if he was thinking of bailing, but he kept his eyes on the crowd. We watched Flip wander into the kitchen, and then it was just us and the gamers on the couch.

It was tense for about a minute; I couldn't imagine running—where would I go?—but the rumble of my survival instinct was rising.

And then, like the rings of smoke, it all just dissipated.

"Waa gwaan, bredren?" one of them said. *What's going on, friend?*

"Sidung." *Come sit down.* He was a wide dude with a black bandanna wrapped around his head, legs spread and taking up like half the couch. Another guy passed over one of the blunts and handed me the PlayStation controller. Just like that, we were absorbed into the scene.

We played a few games of Madden NFL, then Flip returned from a back room. "We gonna do this or what?" he said.

The bulky guy tossed his controller onto the table, shifting one of the guns, and got up. Laurence and I followed him into a back room where he vacuum-sealed the product for us to ship it. We wrapped the bags in fresh T-shirts, boxed them, and mailed the packages back home.

When we got back to our hotel late that night, Laurence and I laughed, both admitting we didn't know how that was going to play out, relieved that nothing exploded on us. But that was the norm— things didn't happen a lot, but the possibility always hovered. You just never knew.

CHAPTER
8

THE WALL

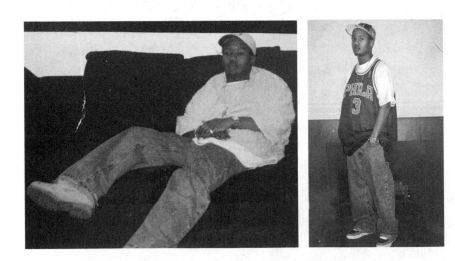

I'D BEEN DEALING FOR ONLY A FEW MONTHS when these pictures were taken at Roc's house. In the first photo I'm wearing a Coogi sweater, a Citizen watch, and a diamond pinky ring, which I'd pawn years later for rent. In the other photo I'm wearing an authentic Mitchell

& Ness throwback Philadelphia 76ers jersey, the same one from the famous Allen Iverson cover of *Slam* magazine where he's all badass with his hair picked out. I got the matching Sixers hat; a pair of custom red, white, and blue Nike Air Force 1s; and a diamond TechnoMarine watch, a half-karat in the bezel. In both pictures I have on a 14-karat white gold necklace with a diamond-encrusted praying hands piece made of 10-karat white gold. I have the same look on my face in both pictures: my fuck-the-world scowl. Like I'm not scared of anything. And for some time, I wasn't.

Soon after my run-in with Jojo, we came back from Tennessee with heroin and people were complaining about the batch. It was grainier than the powder, probably less pure than normal, but it was still legitimate. Customers were trying to get over on us. "This is shit," they'd say. "I need some extra pills or something."

"Fuck no," I'd say.

"This shit is wack. I'm not getting high off it."

"What? That's bullshit," I'd insist. "The shit is official, fam. Fuck outta here."

"I'm telling you, man, this latest was all duds."

When I told Laurence about how this kept happening, he told me to give them a free dose to use in front of me.

"What? I don't want to see that," I said.

He was counting bills at the time and froze, meeting my eyes. "Shit, don't matter what you want to see, man," he said, almost surprised. "This is your livelihood. Your money. You stand there and you watch him."

A few days later another customer, Paul, was trashing my product to me on the phone.

"I want to buy eight hundred worth but that last batch was weak," he said.

"What? That's bullshit."

"If I can't trust the product I gotta go elsewhere. You understand, right?"

He had this false politeness that made my skin crawl.

Not people, a voice said.

"Fuck that," I told him. "Bring your money and equipment and meet me at the carryout place on Caton."

Paul was a goth dude in his twenties, pale and skinny with spiked black hair. He had a stud in his nose and piercings around the perimeter of both ears. Everything he wore was black: jeans, T-shirt, steel-toe boots. He was very timid, rarely said much, and never hung around for long. He spoke monotone with his head down and never made eye contact. Paul was basically a shady guy who used civility as a cover.

We met up at the carryout, a greasy local place I'd spent many hours in. Paul followed me into the dingy bathroom stall, sat down on the closed toilet, and took out his needle, a spoon, and lighter. Then, he got out a cotton ball and a belt to tie around his arm. I had never seen someone shoot up close like that and I wanted like all hell to get out of there. Paul sensed the tension and got nervous. He started fumbling with his setup. "Sorry, the syringe is not working right," he said.

"Enough of this shit, man," I said, leaning against the stall door. "I don't wanna be here. Shoot it or give me ten dollars for the pill you just wasted."

"All right, sorry. Hold on. I'm almost there."

He sprinkled the grainy powder on the spoon, put a bit of water in the syringe, and squeezed it onto the powder. He held a lighter under it until it turned dark brown and looked like tar. He put the cotton ball on top of the spoon to extract the heroin, then pressed the needle into his arm. When he pulled the needle plunger back, it took out some blood, washed red and cloudy, then he pushed back in.

Immediately, his eyes rolled back and he slumped, limp. He started smacking his lips like he was tasting it and just hung there, like his muscles had been extracted. Every time he tried to open his eyes, they'd close right back, like he was fighting sleep.

"So what's up?" I said. "We good?"

He was nodding in and out, his head wobbling. I had my answer. I took what he owed me out of his pocket and tossed the package of pills on his lap. Once I got out of the bathroom, I had to fight the urge to throw up.

Watching Paul in that dirty stall was like a form of self-punishment, forcing myself to stare at the reality of this thing that I was protected from as a kid. I never connected it to my father at the time, but looking back I do. It was Grandma's basement again, only this time I was there, making it happen.

One of my regular clients was Brian, a doughy black guy with a receding hairline who dressed in dingy clothes and carried a thick smell. He walked like a penguin that'd been shot in the leg. One time he asked for $300 worth of product, but he only had $150 on him.

"Sorry, man," I said, getting back in my car. "Hit me up when you got it all."

He reached for my shoulder. "C'mon, Moe. You know I'm good for it."

"Fuck no," I said, shaking him off. "I don't work on credit."

"How about . . . okay, look, I got food stamps. I get five hundred dollars a month in stamps. How about I give you, like, three hundred of that?"

"I don't need groceries," I said. Junkies were always trying to negotiate like that. I had a client at the time whose husband was a hunter. She was hell-bent on trying to offer me pounds of deer meat instead of money.

"C'mon, help me out, man," Brian said.

"I'm not here to help you out, homeboy," I said.

"Shi-i-it," he said. He got almost twitchy. Laurence's words found their target. They weren't people anymore. They were just means to an end.

"Okay," I said. "I'll take the stamps, but I want all of it. All five hundred."

"Can't do that, man. This is all I have for the month. I gotta feed my family. C'mon—"

"Not my problem," I said, starting my car. "You should have thought about that before you offered it."

"But we won't be able to eat," he pleaded.

"Don't give me that shit. That doesn't concern me. You want it or not?"

He caved.

I trailed him out to the Giant grocery store a few blocks down. When we got there, I grabbed a shopping cart and had him follow me as I pulled all the big-ticket items: pork tenderloins, expensive cuts of steak, lobster tails, snow crab legs. I started planning a feast. He had this nervous energy, clearly desperate for his hit.

When I got home, it was like Christmas. That night we invited Christina's parents over for dinner and cooked up some tenderloin and lobster. They were impressed. "Where are you getting this money from?" her mother asked.

"Quentin hit his goal at work," Christina said. "He got a monthly bonus."

"Nice work," her dad said.

"Good for you, Quentin," her mom said.

Things got pretty deep in those years with Laurence. I started carrying around a blue .380 handgun, which I'd stash under the driver's seat anytime I went out. In my apartment I had money hidden inside the vents and behind the walls. I ripped up the carpet and floorboards and hid stacks of money wrapped in rubber bands under there. I wrapped heroin in a black plastic bag and stashed it underneath my stove, taped up and covered in Vaseline to throw off police dogs. After a customer of mine got pinched, he called me and said the police were preparing to raid my house. I got everything out of the house and buried it in my backyard until I could find a new hiding spot.

When I came home at the end of the day or night to Christina, it was never about how my day was. She didn't seem to care about the risk I was running to provide for us. We were making so much money that she could stay home all day and buy stuff off the Home Shopping Network and QVC. That was her life. She knew what I was up to—our apartment was drowning in evidence. During a heroin drought I got into selling crack, which I didn't really know how to make. I bought the cocaine and cooked it up on the stove in my kitchen. Christina came through once while she was talking on the phone. She got annoyed when she saw me. "You're scraping up our pot, Q," she said, covering the mouthpiece. "You gotta use something else." Then she walked out.

Things came into focus for me one Valentine's Day. I had thousands in cash in my pocket and I was going to take Christina on a shopping spree. To set the scene for the reveal, I bought her balloons and candy. "Uh, thank you," she said, all agitated.

"What's your problem?"

"I don't want this shit, Quentin. What're you, in junior high school?"

"What?" I was dumbfounded.

"I know what you make, Quentin. It's Valentine's Day. I was expecting some clothes, or like a Coach bag. Jewelry from Littman's. Not fucking balloons."

Her reaction that day was like a hammer smashing the façade. I canceled the whole shopping idea and went out for a drive, realizing she was more in love with what I could do for her than with me. Young, stubborn, and unwilling to let go of our egos, we were just a ticking clock after that. As I sank further into the game, Christina and I grew apart. We broke up shortly thereafter, and I lived anywhere I could. I'd still sleep there occasionally, but I'd also sleep at Uncle Jason's apartment, in my car, or a hotel.

My mother was working as a manager at a clothing store, and I'd regularly stop in to see her. One of the employees was a cute girl a few years younger than me: slim built and fresh faced, with a radiance that lit up even the bleak fluorescent store. But she dressed like an Amish girl, draped in these ratty long dresses with flower patterns. I went up and introduced myself one day and she told me her name was Tamia. She was a college student working part-time for my mom.

I was booming with confidence in those days—making more money than just about anyone I knew, a success for the first time in my life. At the end of our conversation, I told Tamia, "Well, whenever you're ready I'll take you out shopping. Get you some better clothes." She laughed me off but I kept at it. "C'mon girl, let me take you out. These dresses are not working for you." She accepted it, almost like a dare, to see if I'd go through with it.

When I took her out, she started asking questions about where I got my money, and I just told her that I owned my own business. I tended to go low-key in my dress, and because she knew my mother, she didn't think I was in the streets. I didn't drive a fancy car, and in my day-to-day, I often wore sweatpants, a black hoodie, and dusty Timberlands.

The next time I saw Tamia at the store, she asked something that nobody had ever asked me before. When I walked in, she said, "How was your day?" I stopped cold. It was a simple thing, but it stamped an impression on me because in years, Christina never did that even once. Besides that kindness, Tamia had the air of someone who wanted something more out of life, as did I.

I was coming out of many years of people writing me off, and now was taking care of my business, more confident than I ever was, a success on anyone's terms. Growing up poor set the standards for me. Being able to buy certain things gave me a sense of power, independence, and pride. It wasn't about the money; it was about the importance that I felt from having the money. It was also the feeling of mastery and confidence that comes with being good at something. But I flew full speed past confidence into arrogance.

It was not until we got serious that Tamia even knew I was dealing. She was curious, so she might have suspected, but it wasn't confirmed until I had to make a last-minute deal one day with her in the car. She sat and waited and when I got back in the car, there was no hiding it. We had crossed that threshold. It actually brought us closer because there were no more walls between us. She knew that I trusted her enough to open the curtain on that part of my life.

When Tamia got pregnant about a year later, I had to reevaluate what I was doing. I started to think hard about getting out of the game, but it wasn't an easy task; I was caught up in the fast money. By this time I had stopped selling to local addicts and started selling in bulk to suppliers, people coming from Pennsylvania and Virginia, guys who bought $3,000 worth every 2 or 3 days.

One night I was in my car at my meet-up spot, a restaurant parking lot, waiting on a customer. I was zoned out, listening to old-school hip-hop on the radio. A group of guys strolled over to my car. One of them knocked on my window and I rolled it down.

"Fam, you can't be here."

"What are you talking about?" I asked.

"You making the spot hot," he said. "If you ain't from round here, you can't eat here."

"I'm from just up the way—"

He leaned toward my window, putting his face closer to me. "Main man, if we see you round here again, we gon' have a problem."

"I hear you," I said, slowly reaching my hand underneath my seat. I didn't think it would escalate to me needing my pistol, but you never knew: It didn't hurt to prepare. "But the people that I'm hitting ain't even from around here."

"Don't matter. You making it hot for all of us. I don't wanna see you around here no more." With that, they all walked off.

Two nights later, I was back. I didn't take them seriously; I was in my own mind. After I finished a deal with a customer, I started crossing the lot back to my car. Right as I opened the door, I heard, "That's yo right there." Under the streetlights I saw some figures approaching. Then I heard a *click clack*, the sound of pistols being cocked, and I just took off. When I looked back, I saw four or five guys rushing at me. I crossed over the main street and lit out.

Shots were fired somewhere behind me, once, then twice. A piercing echo through the night as my heart went jackrabbit. I ran full speed down the sidewalk, booking down to the only lights I saw in the distance: St. Agnes Hospital. When I got there, I popped into the emergency room and waited them out. After an hour or so, they scattered. That incident put some real fear into me, shook me from my foundation.

Then came the final straw.

Phil was a small-time local dealer I had known for some time. Word had gotten out that he'd been arrested and he disappeared for a short while. Then he rang me up late one night out of the blue.

"Yo, Moe," he said. "I need you to help me out. This is my last order. I need like ten pounds by tonight. You can hook me up?"

Something wasn't right. It was an extremely large request, his tone was jittery, and the phone was echoing like there was a bug on the line.

"Who is this?"

"It's Phil, man. C'mon, Moe. I know you still with Laurence. This is going to be my last order, I just need—"

"Sorry, sir, there's no Moe here," I said. "I don't know a Laurence. You have the wrong number."

"Shit, I know what you'd been hearing about the cops," he said. "It's bullshit. I just really need you to come through for me."

"I don't know who you are but you're talking pretty reckless on the phone. I don't know you. Please don't call me again. I'm sleeping here with my family." As I hung up the phone, I thought, *I'm done*. God was laying it out for me: now or never. The inevitable end of every drug dealer was never clearer to me than at that point.

Turns out that Laurence had come to the same conclusion. "Yo," he said. "I'm going to do a couple more runs and I'm done."

"I'm with you," I said. We came to a mutual agreement, like a pact. We were like family, and we both knew that it wasn't worth it anymore.

When I first started with Laurence, I had ambitions of taking over the operation. But between the shooting, the setup, and the child on the way, the allure of the streets started to sour. The life started to reveal itself for what it really was; I was fighting a battle that no one ever wins. Things were bound to play out badly. I was going to be killed or imprisoned. The fear of what that would look like—what my mom would think—was a huge influence on my decision. The street was catching up to me, getting ready to crash into me at full speed.

Memories of my father also played a role. I didn't want my unborn child, through no fault of his own, to experience what I went through. Pop was addicted to using drugs, and I was addicted to selling them. But we would've been the same, and I'd have no one to blame but myself. I would perpetuate the cycle, have my own son resenting me deep into his adulthood. It just wasn't worth it.

Christian was born on a cold January day about 6 months later. I held his tiny body in the hospital and stared into his unfocused eyes while Tamia rested beside us. The decision to drop the street life took no effort; it was easy to leave it all behind. It flowed out of me as naturally as lifting my son.

CHAPTER
9

THE FALL

CHRISTIAN HAD THIS JOVIAL INNOCENCE that I never got tired of, lighting up rooms and filling my heart. Before he was even 2 years old, he was something of a performer, reminding me of myself popping and locking like Michael Jackson. We'd all be in church listening intently and I'd notice Christian out of the corner of my eye. He'd hop off his mother's lap and stand in front of his seat, mimicking the pastor, gesturing electrically with his little arms and hands. The pastor of my church was a world-renowned preacher, Dr. Jamal Harrison Bryant of the Empowerment Temple. He was an energetic man and powerful speaker with a deep gravel growl of a voice. Christian wasn't mimicking him to be funny; it was no different than a child imitating a superhero, but it was hilarious to watch. Everyone in our section would be busting up laughing while nearby pews eyed and shushed us.

Chris's arrival made me come to terms with what kind of family I wanted him to have. What kind of things I could rewrite and revise this time around. I didn't want my own issues with family to limit the reach and scope of his life. My father had been out of prison for years by this point, had cleaned up, and was living in an apartment with his new wife and baby daughter around the corner from us. He was working two jobs, had put on pounds, and toned down in temperament. With time, especially after leaving the drug game, my own intense feelings about him dissipated. I made a conscious decision to let my father be a part of Chris's life, having him over to the house regularly—reestablishing our relationship and hoping he'd develop one with my son.

I found a job working in automotive sales. A neighbor of mine was the manager of a car dealership and hired me as a new car salesman. The huge drop in income at the simultaneous arrival of another mouth to feed was substantial, like a change in air pressure. Roc would call from time to time and it was clear he was on an upward trajectory. He was progressing to kingpin status, moving kilos of heroin at a time out of a place not far from my grandmother's house. "Yo, Q," he said on the phone about 6 months after I had quit. "Come check out my operation, meet some people, see what we got going on here."

"Nah," I told him. "Definitely appreciate it, but I'm out. I'm good."

"Just come by," Roc said. "Let me show you my new operation. I got a place for you, man. It's solid."

"Well, you know you're my man, but I'm out. Like out-out."

"I hear you, Moe, I hear you," he said. Roc and I had a long and tested bond. I had a feeling his persistence in reaching out meant he must've needed me. As he was expanding, he likely needed someone close to him, someone whose trust was unquestionable. "Well, just think about it," he said. "I'll put you on with some people, show you that it's all good."

I was tempted, and felt strange saying no to him, like forcing my muscles to bend a new way. He sensed the opening.

"How about you just swing by?" he proposed. "Just chill."

"All right," I said. "I'll slide through."

Going straight was like pushing a rock uphill that kept tumbling back down over me. I had cycled through a few different jobs—collections agent, jewelry store associate, credit card salesman. Each time I had to adjust to a new lifestyle, daily structure, and skill set. When I stopped by Roc's place a few nights later, I might have been unconsciously primed. I got lost in a longer conversation with him about getting back in. Then he made me a direct offer.

"Okay, how 'bout this?" he said, feeling my give. "How 'bout you do a trip for me?"

"Trip? What kind of trip?"

"Next week. Drive down to Greensboro, make a pickup for me, and I'll give you fifteen K."

Fifteen thousand dollars for 8 hours in a car. I had promised Tamia and myself that I was done, but it felt irresponsible turning down that kind of money. And I could rationalize it because Roc presented it like it'd be a one-time thing. I could use that stake to start a business, I thought. Get out of the rut that had me awake at night, wondering how I'd support my family.

I said yes.

A few days later, Tamia was out and I was on the floor playing with Chris. He was rolling around, and I was tickling his belly. In the stillness of the room, with just the sound of his laugh, I realized I was lying to myself. There was no such thing as a one-time deal. This job would snowball to the next and before I knew it, I'd be a cog in the operation. It was a natural progression. Like any other addiction, in order to stay clean you need to abstain from it. The thrill of a taste could easily trap me.

I grabbed the phone and dialed Roc: I couldn't do it. He had to find someone else. He was understanding, still open to the fact that I'd come around. "No problem, Moe," he said. "It's all good."

"Appreciate you looking out, though," I said.

"Remember, whatever you need, I got you. Come fuck with me. You know how we roll."

"I know it."

About a month later, Roc rang me up and invited me over on a Saturday night. It was unspoken that maybe we'd discuss work, again getting me into his operation.

"Why don't you come out tonight? We can just trip."

"Nah, I can't," I said. "Soon though."

"Come on, yo. It's real chill tonight," he said. "Not too much popping off."

"I told Shorty I would chill with her tonight. We'll meet up in a couple of days though, for sure."

"I feel you. Can't disappoint wifey," he said. "It's all good. Just get at me tomorrow."

The next morning in church, I heard whispers floating through the crowd. The night before, Roc was outside a house in Park Heights, conversing with another dealer about territory, going over discrepancies about who controlled which corner. After a few minutes, they came to an agreement; no threats made, no arguing, nothing in the air that usually precedes violence. But as Roc was walking away, one of the guys who'd been standing around pulled out a gun and started firing at Roc, hitting him in the head, lower back, and arm. He lay sprawled on the pavement, and everyone scattered.

I sat frozen in the aisle, first floored by the shock of it, then swarmed by a heavy sense of guilt. I fell to my knees. The tears just flowed out. I should've been there with him. Maybe I would've gotten him out of there in time, would've known what was shaky, who couldn't be trusted. It was wishful thinking, but I had proven instincts: I'd never been shot, was never picked up by the cops, and had good luck during my time in the game.

Roc lay in a coma at the hospital, and I visited him practically every day. When he came out of it about a month later, he had lost his sight and could barely communicate; he was only able to move his fingers to respond. Nine months later, he was released from the hospital, able to see but paralyzed for life on his right side. He had always been such a vibrant presence, joyful and larger than life—seeing him like that was like a hole cut in the world. In a lot of ways, I feel like Roc's life was sacrificed to save mine. Had that not happened to him, I very likely would've gotten back into the drug game eventually. There were too many temptations, too many opportunities, and too much money to keep walking away from. But his lifeless body in the hospital bed, then the version of himself that emerged, offered a stark message.

I slammed the door shut on that life, bolted it, and walked away for good.

Life at home with Tamia got more and more hectic. Our money issues exacerbated other things that had been lingering under the surface. We both loved Christian and wanted to be the best parents we could, but the strain between us was undeniable. We were both very young—I was only 23, Tamia was 21—as well as hotheaded and bull stubborn. In some ways we mirrored my parents' relationship. There was never any violence, but our youth, inexperience, and competing desires just rippled into everything. They ate up the best of our intentions and eroded our genuine feelings. It reached a breaking point: For everyone's sanity and livelihood, we agreed to separate.

The morning after we came to this decision, my father was at the house in an attempt to mediate the situation. Tamia was packing her things and told my father privately that I was "kicking her out." My father came over to me while I was sitting in the living room.

"Quentin, I don't know what—"

"You promised me we'd always be together," Tamia yelled from the bedroom, "and you'd always be there for me!"

My father ran with it, suddenly a model dispenser of justice. "You're supposed to be a man, son," he said to me. "And you're supposed to take care of your family no matter what! You can't just kick this girl out; she's telling me that—"

"You don't even know what you're talking about!" I shot back. I was furious. Not just at how wrong the message was, but the gall of the messenger. "You got some nerve coming at me! You haven't honored your commitment since I was seven years old." I told him he was the last father in the world who could give out this kind of scolding.

He flipped, cut in the way that only the truth can cut you. "You're not going to disrespect me; I'm still your father."

"The fuck you are! You just some guy who had sex with my mother! You feel that strongly, you let her stay with you!"

He grabbed me and slammed me against the wall, and we started shoving and tussling until Tamia's screaming made us stop. I stormed out of the house and went for a walk, my anger coursing through my blood, my adrenaline spiked for hours afterward. Once I'd calmed down, the tears flowed out of me, the frustration a palpable force. I closed the door again on my relationship with my father, tired of letting this man back into my life, sick of giving him a free pass to disappoint me again and again. The most infuriating part was that nothing had changed; he still didn't know me at all.

Tamia and I had spoken frequently about raising Christian together outside Baltimore. It rose from our desire for him to have more, to experience something different than we had. We hadn't even yet discussed how to handle custody with our breakup when she said she wanted to take him down to Florida. She said she had a job offer and could live near her family down there.

An instinct rose up inside me: I would not let my son go. I'd fight tooth and nail to keep him with me and make sure he had the father in his life that I never had. I knew firsthand how important that was.

But I was naive. I met with a lawyer and it became clear that the court system's setup would make it a losing battle. The burden is on the father to prove a mother is unfit; a mother doesn't have to do anything but just be. There was no court in America that was going to give me custody of my son.

There were months of back and forth, and I reached a point where I knew I was prolonging the inevitable. I couldn't rationalize more court dates and more lawyer fees, making it even harder on Chris, who was slowly becoming aware of what was going on. It would've damaged him emotionally, which is exactly what I was trying to prevent. So I stopped fighting.

Months later, on a hot summer day, Tamia and I were in a cramped room at the Baltimore City Courthouse with a mediator, a short, blonde white woman in her forties. We all sat at a dark wooden table and my eyes scanned the bulletin boards with pinned notices on the dirty eggnog walls. The air conditioner was on full blast, loud and rattling, a sharp contrast to the thick summer heat but its own kind of stifling.

Agreeing to the terms the court set forth—allowing Tamia to take Christian a thousand miles away—was like tearing a piece of myself from my body. I tried to justify it all, told myself he'd have a better standard of living, better schools, a safer situation in Florida. Who was I to put a ceiling and walls around him so early, hinder what he could become? Letting go was only possible if I told myself these things.

After Tamia and Chris's departure, things got particularly dark and difficult for me. She would e-mail pictures of Chris and each change in his face, each milestone, was like a blow to the chest. He was at the age where even a week made a visible difference; his childhood was slipping through my fingers. The pictures were almost too hard to look at and just reinforced the feeling that I'd made the biggest mistake of my life. They'd be up to Baltimore for Christmas vacation, and I had mandatory visitation every spring break and summer break, but it was like a slow, agonizing drip. It just wasn't enough, and it only magnified what I was missing. I felt like I had done the one thing I had vowed not to do: fail as a father. Alcohol became my medication, cigarettes my coping mechanism. But everything I did to ease the pain only made it worse; it all just dug me deeper.

Soon after, I got fired from my job as a car salesman and had to move back in with my mother. It was a serious blow to my pride, out of which grew an all-consuming depression, like a heavy cloud settling around me. The loneliness started closing in on me, and nothing I did gave me space to breathe. The only times I would leave the house would be to buy alcohol and cigarettes at the liquor store across the street and when I would go to the gym.

I started to take exercising seriously in a way I never had before, trying to work my way out of my depression.

At 5' 7" and a spindly 130 pounds, I'd always had body image issues, which swelled into self-esteem issues. Sometimes they were at the forefront of my mind, sometimes they were a nagging voice in the background. I was plagued by my idea of what women viewed as a "real man:" tall, muscular, physically strong. Everything I wasn't. Because there was nothing I could do about my height, I lifted heavy weights five times a week trying to change everything else.

My drinking would always be at night, occasionally alone in the afternoon. I would buy a half-pint of Hennessy or Jack Daniels, sit at home in my bedroom, and drink. I'd be smoking cigarette after cigarette, pouring glass after glass.

I was living a contradiction, a tidy ball of self-negation, building up my body while simultaneously destroying it. It was like picking myself up and then dropping myself from an increasingly greater height.

<hr />

During the breakdown of my relationship with Tamia, I had to throw on a tux and serve as best man at a friend's wedding in Atlanta. I was too loyal a friend to back out, and I had to drag myself around every movement that weekend. I used his wedding weekend as an excuse to drink even more. From the time I got off the plane, I had a drink in my hand. It was an out-of-body experience, my world back home crumbling, and I was an apparition of myself, going through the motions.

During the rehearsal I started talking to one of the bridesmaids, Nicole, a New Jersey girl a few years younger than me. She was short, very slim, and beautiful, with an intoxicating laugh. We shared a few dances at the reception, and afterward chatted at the dais. Our joking took a natural turn to the serious when she opened up about a difficult relationship she was in. I kept my issues to myself, but I tried to give her some advice. At the end of the weekend, I told her we should try to be in touch.

"Hey, we're family now," I told her. "I'ma be looking out for you. Whether you like it or not."

About 4 or 5 months after that wedding, after Tamia and Chris had moved out, Nicole and I reconnected online. I was spending a lot more time home alone, drinking myself into a stupor, and messing around on the computer until the quiet hours of the night. Our posts evolved into texts and then phone calls, and soon we were talking for hours every night. She talked to me about trying to extract herself from her relationship and I listened, and I offered advice when it seemed warranted. Then I started to trust her and opened up about my own feelings of failure regarding my son, my broken relationships, and the pain of my childhood.

By this point, the drinking was center stage in my life. It had shifted from a strictly nighttime thing to an occasional afternoon thing to a morning routine and everything after thing. The line kept moving earlier and earlier into the day until there was no distinction from the night before. It was the haze I carried to face the world, the armor I wore to face myself. I was an emotional mess: caught in a loop, impossible to talk to, and shut off from the world. I had regressed to a childhood self, angry and closed off. Living at my mother's just added to the feeling that I had been stripped, roughed up, and dropped back into adolescence.

"I don't know if I can make it anymore," I told Nicole on the phone one night, bleary-eyed and lying down on my bed. "Shit's too hard. Maybe . . . maybe Chris is better off without me." Part of me meant it, part of me was saying it just to feel what crossing that line felt like. My face was pressed to the bottom.

I stared at the giant gray television on mute, headlines crawling across the bottom of the screen and circling back around again. The words a foreign language, the newscaster's face an alien. My eyes drifted to the rickety brown console, my baseball caps on nails on the wall above.

"Don't talk like that!" she said. "Your son needs his father."

"Not if this is what his father is!"

I was chain-smoking Marlboro Menthols and drinking bourbon straight out of a cloudy highball glass, the ashtray collecting into a bleak sculpture. The window was open onto the back alley, to a silent night, nothing but the faint sound of a dog's yelp.

"God doesn't disappear," she said, firm and calm. "He didn't bring you this far to leave you now."

An engine revved and pulsated a few blocks over, a growling animal in the night.

"Quentin? Quentin, you there?"

"I'm here."

"I said, it's not random. There's a reason why we met," she said—*wise beyond her age,* I thought. "I'm here for you."

"I can't imagine why."

"You let me worry about that," she said, a light laugh in her voice.

For reasons that could only be attributed to grace, Nicole stuck around. She'd call me every day to see how my day had gone, and she put up with fluctuations in mood and tone and temperament that I'd wish on no one. She even drove from Jersey to Baltimore one Friday evening to surprise me and check up on me. After a gesture like that, I knew enough to hold on tight. Then, I used her sturdiness to pull myself up enough to stand.

It was a slow process, but I cut back on drinking and got a job working as a used car salesman. Nicole's visits continued, our relationship got serious, then one day she told me she was pregnant. Though things in my life were rough, the news brought me joy. There was a sense of solidity to Nicole, which somehow helped bind me to the future.

CHAPTER
10

STRANGER

WITH A TWO-BEDROOM APARTMENT IN THE BALTIMORE SUBURBS, a loving woman, and a newborn son, I was relaunched. An energy began to flow through me as I took things head-on, confident and eager to succeed. Back into life.

Jayden was the happiest kid on the planet. All he wanted out of life was to eat and dance. We played a lot of music in the house, and when he started crawling, Nicole and I noticed he was drawn to it. We'd be sitting in the living room and he'd be playing with his toys on the floor. When I put on some music through my computer, he'd crawl over to the laptop and start rocking back and forth on his hands and knees. On beat. As if the music were flowing through him.

While Nicole was pregnant, I had buckled down and gotten a license to sell life insurance. Once Jayden was born, I became an insurance rep and began training as a financial planner. At 26, with nothing more than a high school diploma and a few semesters of college, I had a legitimate job and a two-bedroom apartment in Baltimore County. And Tamia had moved back to Baltimore with Christian, so we were doing father-son things together, such as going to the aquarium down by the harbor. I had an unconventional but tightening family. For the first time in a while, I felt as though I had my footing.

But my success, comfort, and loving relationship didn't break my depression. I was still haunted by my mistakes and other failures—the people I hurt and the ones who hurt me. Although I wasn't drinking as much as I had been before Nicole, I was finding new ways to numb these feelings. I smoked close to a pack of cigarettes a day and could easily lose myself in a few bottles of wine on any given night. It became my reward, then my rock, then my normalcy.

The one healthy thing I could turn to was the gym. Working out got me out of my head, away from my problems, and focused me on what I could touch and see. The gym was an open and bright space, with a positive energy flowing through the room. Flat-screen televisions perched above the treadmills, elliptical machines, and bikes. A front area of resistance machines. A large rack of dumbbells on the far wall in front of the group fitness room. The walls were cream with white trim, the mats black rubber, the weight benches a royal blue. Mirrors lined every wall, creating an illusion of a bigger space with more people.

I had become so compulsive about working on my body that I entered a men's physique competition and began to train for it. Just about every day I'd do an hour session, focused entirely on gaining muscle mass by lifting heavy weights: bench press, dumbbell and rear delt flies, curls, military press, tricep pulldowns. It was all about going heavy and increasing my gains. To build mass, I'd start off by drinking a pre-workout supplement and end with an 850-calorie protein shake. I had become so dialed in to the process—such an ecstatic convert to its power—that I began training clients on my own. The gym had become my go-to place, my haven, my sanctuary.

But without warning, the gym turned into a prison, one that originated inside my own body. On a summer afternoon in 2009, a few months after Jayden was born, the world as I knew it was smashed, shattered, and flipped upside down.

I was in the midst of my routine at the gym, doing my bench presses on the incline barbell rack. In the middle of a set, a sharp pain appeared in the left side of my chest. Stirred, I carefully rested the bar in the metal brackets and waited, trying to get a sense of what was happening. When I stood up, I felt lightheaded, like I'd gotten up too quickly and air had been sucked out of my head. Putting my hand on the bench, I folded over to maintain balance. I pressed my fingers against my chest, trying to locate the pain, figuring I just pulled a muscle. I stared at a clock on the far wall, a fixed point, and watched the second hand tick. After about a minute, the feeling dissipated, so I sat back down and continued my set.

By my third rep the pain returned, more persistent, demanding. It was accompanied by this tingling sensation, which started at the fingertips of my left hand and moved up my arm, like a foreboding message squirreling through my body. I put the bar down again and sat up. *This is not normal,* I thought. I took a drink of water and again waited for it to pass. This time, though, fear began bubbling up, even as I tried to talk myself out of it. *If I don't acknowledge it, it's not really there.* But it was creeping fast. Then faster. Then, as I stood up again, it was on me.

My heart picked up speed, rocketed forward and beat furiously, like someone slamming on an accelerator. I checked my heart rate on my watch monitor—150 beats per minute, significantly higher than normal, despite the fact that this was my normal workout. Something about seeing the numbers, the recognition of the facts, sent me into a panic. I started to hyperventilate and the room began spinning, the perimeter mirrors exacerbating the effect.

I have to get home, I thought. *If I make it home—see Nicole—I'll be okay.*

I scrambled outside for sunlight and fresh air, but the chaos of the outside world made it worse. My body felt like putty, and I had to drag myself through the parking lot. I found my car, fumbled with getting out my keys and the suddenly difficult task of opening the door. I let gravity drop me into the driver's seat and took a look at myself in the rearview mirror, trying to reconcile that face with this person. I seemed like a stranger to myself, distant from my limbs, swimming and disoriented. When I tried to throw the car into reverse, I felt intoxicated. I couldn't align my movements with the car's and I pulled the car straight back into the curb. After struggling to repark and get out, I found a bench in front of the strip mall to wait it all out. Nothing was balanced. The blue mailbox on the curb seemed turned on its side. The wooden bench wasn't steady. Everything was in motion.

I'm not going to die, I told myself.

On the bench, my heart rate read 170 beats per minute. But my energy level was draining out of me like a liquid, my arms heavy and my body becoming a lump. It was as though a force was rising from my limbs into my neck, then head. The ground was coming up to meet me, on an angle, like I was going to pass out.

I fumbled for my phone and dialed 911, then moved down to lie on the curb, my arm wrapped around the pole of a street sign.

"I'm having a heart attack," I said the moment I heard the click of someone answering. I couldn't describe it any other way and knew it would cut through with those words. A young woman's tinny voice tried to calm me.

"Okay, stay there. We're going to send help. Where are you?"

"I'm at the shopping center on York and Seminary. In front of the Rite Aid," I told her. "I'm on the curb. I can't move."

"Okay, someone's on the way. Stay there and don't drink anything." Her voice was a faint noise from a distant planet.

"Please hurry up," I begged. "I can't do this much longer."

She started to ask what I had taken and what I had been doing. I was struggling to breathe, much less talk. I tried to imagine each breath going through me. My eyes felt heavy as though I'd been awake for days. My mouth was dry and my body weakening, like air draining from a tire.

I felt trapped inside my own body, like a plane in a tailspin, hurtling toward the earth. I closed my eyes and said a prayer.

Lord God, please let me make it through this.
Allow me to raise my children
To see another day.
Please forgive my wrongdoings and create in me a clean heart . . .
I ask that your will be done
In Jesus' mighty name
Amen.

Then, piercing the thin air, was the high-pitched wail of a siren. I could hear it coming closer, on top of me . . . then flying past.

"They just fucking passed me!" I wheezed out into the phone, the operator's voice still lingering in my hand. "You guys trying to kill me?!"

"Sir, please calm down. I'll have them turn around. Give us the address again."

"I don't know the address! I'm in front of the Rite Aid on Seminary!"

My heart was a wild horse off its stake, trampling forward. I thought of my sons, of Nicole, of my mother. I prayed. Everything slowed to a crawl.

The ambulance finally careened into the parking lot. Two paramedics hopped out and started in on me, rapid-fire.

What's your name, sir?
Do you know what day it is?

What did you take?

Tell us what's wrong.

Sir, can you tell us what's wrong?

"My heart is . . . racing out . . . I can't breathe . . . can't talk." Everything was coming out breathy and stilted, like I'd been pulled from the water.

"Relax, sir. Just try to relax," one of them said, which of course only made me panic more. The other EMT hooked a mask over my mouth to pump oxygen into my system.

He wrapped a black band around my arm and pumped. "Blood pressure's elevated," he said. "Your heart rate is 192 bpm. We have to flush out whatever's in your system."

They put me onto a white stretcher, hooked an IV into my arm, and rushed me into the back of the ambulance.

As we flew through the county streets, my eyes fixed on the metal ceiling, all I could think about was seeing Nicole and my mother. My safety nets. *Just seeing them will level this all out,* I told myself. One of the paramedics called Nicole, who called my mother, who met us at the hospital.

In a tight, brightly lit space in the emergency room, doctors and nurses continued with the IV fluids until my heart rate went down. I felt drained and beaten, an object—talked at, not to.

Some time passed, and my body started to find its rhythm and footing. Then a nurse came by with paperwork and said they were going to release me.

"Wait, what?"

"You're what?" my mother asked simultaneously.

"Doctor's orders," the nurse said with a shrug. "Says you're fine. Probably a caffeine reaction."

"Caffeine?"

"The supplement you take is a testosterone booster. It has caffeine."

"Yeah," I said. "I know." I made eye contact with my mom as we both wordlessly tried to figure out how to protest.

"Plus," she read off the chart, "sixteen ounces of coffee this morning. You had a reaction. It happens."

"But that's normal for me. It's been my routine for over a year. I've been drinking coffee since—"

But she was already throwing the curtain open, on to the next patient. I had been taken off the to-do list, solved.

The next morning, I skipped the gym and had just half a cup of coffee, hoping to erase the previous day's nightmare. But by late morning, it was back. Creeping, then on me. I was caught inside another attack. That night it came on again. Then the next morning.

Then the next.

Then the next.

My body was in a full-blown rebellion. The anxiety started to spread outward, like water seeking any and all cracks. I started to question everything, never feeling grounded or safe. My sleepy neighborhood became a minefield of triggers. As days rolled into weeks, I became too terrified to sleep and too crippled to do anything. I was trapped inside the walls of my own prison.

This was the sequence: My heart would start beating hard, then fast and faster. My mouth would go dry and then I would start to feel dizzy, like the floor was curving upward or I could feel the tilt of the earth. A sensation would start creeping up my left side: fingertips, hand, gaining speed and intensity up my arm and left side.

Then I'd be hit with chest pains, as well as difficulty breathing that usually spiraled into hyperventilation. A powerful force I couldn't see was smothering me. It was like I was at the bottom of a deep hole and dirt was filling in above me.

My own body had become untrustworthy and the world became dangerous. Nicole tried her best to comfort me, but she was as mystified as I was. Watching me obsessively check my heart rate, or seeing me get up in the middle of the night to drive myself to the ER, she felt helpless. It was hard for her to watch this weakened man, scared to be home by himself, always seeking confirmation that he'd be okay. I was a shell of the person she had grown to know and love, as needy as our infant son.

Things got increasingly worse. After waking up in the middle of the night too many times, I started to sleep in my car in the hospital parking lot in case an attack came. I refused to go anywhere that wasn't a quick ride to an emergency room. Walls went up all around me. I was terrified by the loss of control, the inability to predict, the fear of never feeling normal again. I refused to drive long distances and was afraid to work out at the gym, thinking that would keep it at bay. But I still had clients I had to train. I canceled and pushed a few sessions until I had to get back to work. I was secretly afraid of doing even the basic cardio or lifting that I had my clients do. The thing I had once done for peace and strength was now terrifying to me. I often invented injuries or other reasons why I couldn't participate. I'd become a fraud, my life a spectacle.

Sometimes when I'd call 911, an ambulance would arrive, and the attack would dissipate once the paramedics reached me or once I got to the hospital. Once, it just vanished right after I hung up the phone with 911. The appearance—the suggestion—of help would negate its need. This was the first inkling that all of this was from a deeper well.

At the ER, they would hook me up to an IV and give me a sedative to try to induce sleep. Then came countless blood tests, CT scans, and EKGs, but no answers. After every visit the ER doctor would say, "Follow up with your primary," but I didn't have one. About a month into the attacks, I was back at the ER when they gave me a lorazepam pill. It was like a cool breeze blowing through my body. It was a relief. It was magic.

The next morning I finally went to see a general practitioner; I had been putting off the visit for the typical insurance reasons. Dr. Barnes was a tall white guy in his late fifties, with one of those large builds that indicated he had once been heavy. He wore thin-framed glasses, had silver hair along the sides—a bald highway down the middle—and a trimmed beard.

Dr. Barnes looked over the stack of paperwork—all of my blood work, tests, and medical records from all the emergency room visits. I cycled through the explanation of symptoms yet again, which I hated doing because it was like unlocking the cage. An aura of panic floated into the room just by me saying some of those words.

During my recitation of stories and symptoms, he cut me off, putting his hand up. "Okay, Quentin," he said in his nasal voice. "It sounds to me like you have a severe anxiety disorder."

"A disorder?" I asked, confounded. "You mean like a disease?"

"Yes. It's very common. It's called generalized anxiety and panic disorder." I told him about the lorazepam I'd gotten from the hospital, and he prescribed it for me as a daily medicine. I rarely took medicine as a child and vividly remembered my mother's refusal to medicate me as a teenager in the psychiatrist's office. She knew the dangers associated with it a lot more than the average person because she was med certified and had worked in the industry for 25 years.

There was also a cultural divide. There was not a single kid on medication for behavior in my community. One of my cousins was hyperactive; he was the only kid I knew who took medicine to calm down. I knew some diabetics, but that was it. No one took anything for anything.

But what choice did I have? I was a drowning man and the doctor had pulled up in a boat. I put my complete trust in my physician's hands, relieved to know that my problem had a name and that the symptoms were treatable.

"How long do I have to take this?" I asked, staring at the prescription sheet. A strange mix of relief and suspicion weaved through me.

"Well, the disorder is quite severe," he said. "Medication is the only option effective enough to control your anxiety."

He didn't really answer my question, but I didn't push him. I was just happy to have some weapon to fight back.

CHAPTER
11

CRUTCH

LORAZEPAM PULLED ME OUT OF A BURNING BUILDING. I wouldn't go anywhere without my pills, the buoy that I clung to, the magic that had given me myself back.

But it wasn't a self that I wanted to be.

In the months following my diagnosis, the lorazepam worked well. Too well. So well that I used it to patch each and every hole in my life.

The human body adjusts to any medication, so in order to reach the same sense of normalcy, 2 milligrams turned into 4, then into 6 and 8 within a 24-hour period. Then higher. I was forever chasing that feeling of calm and equilibrium. I never trusted that my body would find normalcy on its own. That's the nature of being an addict: You're chasing a thing that is harder and harder to get. You're seeking something that is constantly fleeting.

I carried the pills everywhere, compulsively patting pockets and checking bags to be double and triple sure they were there. I kept a bottle in the medicine cabinet, one in the armrest in my car, some in a Ziploc bag in my gym bag, more inside a folded tissue in my wallet.

My entire approach was preemptive and preventive. I was the beekeeper slipping on the white suit, taking a pill before an attack could even sense an opening. In hindsight, it's strange how complete my reversal was: 26 years with virtually no medication—an aversion to it, really—to then an inability to even conceive of a few hours without it. That's what fear will do to you. The fear of losing control of my body, my footing, my sense of self in the world. I had no interest in even trying to push through the fear to see if I could control it myself; it'd be like jumping out of the plane without a parachute just to feel myself fall to earth. The pills first helped, then overtook who I was, then subsumed me entirely. My logic felt airtight: I hadn't had a single panic attack since the day I had started on them.

And that's how it happened. In the process of wanting to feel safe, to incubate myself from fear, I became an addict.

Not that I noticed it. Even though I grew up around addicts, I didn't realize I had become one. I felt I was just following doctor's orders, taking a medication on a progression. I had a problem, and these small white pills were the solution. In my mind, it was no different than taking blood pressure medication. Because of my mother and the world I grew up in, I had little experience with or exposure to prescription drugs. I was naive and desperate, a particularly dangerous combination.

My doctor never made me feel any different.

"I need you to increase the dosage," I'd say. "I feel like it's weakening. Not working like it should."

"Sure thing," he'd say. "But I can't increase the recommended dose. I'll just write you a script for more pills and you take them as needed."

"Okay. So I just take them until I run out?"

"Correct. I'll write you a script for 120 instead of 60. You can increase the dose and it'll last the same amount of time."

"Okay, cool."

People around me knew what was going on, what had happened, and how I was treating it. I'd go out with friends and if I had stretched it out a few hours without a pill, I might get a little agitated. It wasn't even anxiety; it was just the chemical leaving my body, the perceptible decrease in my bloodstream.

"Quentin, did you take your pill?" Nicole would ask. "You're kind of crabby right now." Or my mother would say, "I think you maybe need to take your medicine, honey."

It's not like I was a robot; I could still get upset, could still disagree. But the minute I did, I always heard: "Have you been taking your medicine? You need to take a pill and chill out." No one knew how often I took them, or how dependent I was. To them, my pills made me a pleasure to be around. It started to become: *You need to take these because we don't like who you are without them.*

I got the message.

After my diagnosis, Dr. Barnes told me that I would likely need to be on medication for the rest of my life. He was unequivocal about it, but he said it like it was no problem. His mind-set seemed to mirror mine: I had attacks, the pills stopped them—problem solved. I could now live a normal, sustainable life.

He never told me, as I later learned, that lorazepam is not a long-term solution at all. It's known for being addictive and for lessening effects over time. The only thing he did say was to stay away from caffeine: no coffee, no pre-workout drinks, no chocolate. At the time, it seemed a small price to pay for having control over myself again.

||||||||||||||||||||||||||||||||||||||||||||||||||||||||||||||||||||||||||||||||||||||

For almost a year after that first attack, the lorazepam let me coast. Things with Nicole were good; Jayden was almost 2, cared for and happy; even my father and I had made amends since our last blowout. I had left finance and was running my own personal training business full time. I signed a coaching contract with a gym in the neighborhood to help train their members. Business was growing and I was in the process of opening my own studio with a partner in Baltimore. We had investors, a business proposal, even a site picked out where we were going to offer cross-training, one-on-one personal training, and spin classes. With magic pills and confidence, a new positivity emerged in my life. I put things out in the world and the world provided back.

As a trainer, I liked to deeply explore my clients' motivations. In our consultations, I would dig into their reasons for working out, why they felt like they couldn't do it, how to persuade them they could. I avoided the sergeant tactics for a more soft-spoken and positive approach. Direct and stern, but personal.

If they said, "I want to lose ten pounds," I'd dig into why.

Some clients would come to me and say, "I'm really looking to get in shape, tone up."

"Is there a specific goal?" I'd push.

"Lose weight. Look better."

"Why?"

"I'm overweight and I don't like the way my arms look."

"That's great, but that's just vanity. That will only take you so far. Why do you really want to lose it? What is your why?" Sometimes they got it right away and we were off. Other times they were more guarded, so I'd push further: Are you afraid you're not going to be here long enough to raise your children? Is there a history in your family you want to fend off? Wanting a six-pack or to look good in a bikini is just not enough.

The vast majority of my private clients were females in their thirties or early forties, young mothers trying to change their habits, confronting their new realities.

I'd train my clients at their homes or at the rec center in Randallstown, a mostly black suburb in the county where I also held classes for about 10 to 15 people at a time. The classes were usually high-intensity intervals and bodyweight exercises—squats, burpees, squat jumps, lunges, jumping jacks, all consecutively. It was an intense 45 minutes. We'd end each class with a cooldown.

One particular day during cooldown at the rec center, everyone was lying down on mats in a cordoned-off section by the indoor track. The class was doing lower back twists. I demonstrated, then walked around to assist members of the group, all lying on their backs, knees together, legs bent in a tabletop position. "Knees to the right, gaze to the left," I said. "Hold it. Don't forget to breathe." Then we switched to the opposite way.

"Great job today, everyone," I said as we wrapped up. "Honor yourselves and the work you just put in. You could've been anywhere in the world but you're here bettering yourselves." I tried to let motivation or even inspirational ideas seep into the workout.

It was a crowded Saturday, two full basketball courts, other coaches yelling, balls bouncing on the floor, voices carrying in the large room, everything echoing off the walls and high ceiling. The noise was at full tilt.

The class dispersed and I reached down to my gym bag. Just as I did I felt a pulse in my right temple and then, like a flipped switch, a persistent throbbing in that spot. It was a clench on my brain, sudden and sharp. I instinctively grabbed my temple and sat down on the floor.

The pain then pressed further inward, pushing behind my eyes, like someone was pressing them back into my skull. The pressure got so intense it was like my brain was being crushed in a vise. I held my head with both hands and stared at the floor until it passed. After an agonizing 10 minutes, I carefully stood up and drove home. I was concerned, took an extra lorazepam to ease my reaction, but I tried not to think too much about it.

Within a few days, the headaches colonized my brain. They became worse, ate up and swallowed whole afternoons. I'd get an aura that one was coming on and I'd find a quiet, dark spot to wait it out. I'd be incapacitated for hours, lying down in a dark room because the light would pierce through my skull. Any noise was a drill boring into the side of my head.

By the third week my vision began to blur along with the headaches, which lifted things to an alarming level. I tried to wave her off but Nicole insisted and drove me to the hospital. I got out of the car, my charcoal gray skullcap pulled down over my eyes and Nicole escorting me through the emergency room. A hospital is like a stage show of bright, fluorescent light. They drew blood, did tests, and gave me a CT scan, but found nothing out of the ordinary. The weight of the world was pushing down on my skull but no one knew why.

In a dimly lit room in the ER, a male nurse trial-and-errored various meds straight through my IV, some kind of painkillers, none of which worked.

"How are you feeling?" he asked after the last attempt. My skullcap was still pulled over my eyes so I didn't get a look at him. He had a deep voice and too casual a manner.

"Not good, man."

"Really?"

"Yeah. The pain is not subsiding in any way," I said into the darkness, the feel of Nicole's hand my only tie to the world. "I'm terrified, to be honest. It's excruciating. Seriously fucking excruciating."

"That bad, huh? Okay, I'll be right back." He left and came back, pushing something new into my IV. "Okay, you're going to feel a rush."

An icy sensation whooshed through my veins and flooded my body. It was intense, like my blood had frozen, and my body chilled from head to toe. My stomach fell to my feet and a wave of nausea took over. A bitter taste washed over my tongue, and I instinctively smacked my lips, able to taste it. That cold flush was overwhelming and spun me into a panic.

"Dude, relax," the nurse said. "Calm down."

"Calm down?!" My heart rate was astronomical. "I'm having a panic attack right now." Nicole started to talk over me, trying to explain my condition and I started yelling about finding me a lorazepam.

"Wait, do you have anxiety or something?" he asked.

"Dude!" I said, agitated, "If you look at the fucking chart, you'll see that I have an anxiety disorder!"

"Oh my God," he said. "I'm so sorry. I just gave you two milliliters of morphine."

Soon after that, the panic was muscled out by the narcotic. I was submerged in a pool of intense calm, but it was too much, shutting out the lights in my brain and turning me into the zombie my mother always railed against me becoming.

At my discharge, the male nurse sat down across from me, still apologetic.

"This is Vicodin," he said. "This will help. It's one of the only prescriptions you can take in conjunction with your anxiety meds without side effects."

Vicodin is a powerful and addictive narcotic, but the ER staff was unaware of my burgeoning addiction and didn't ask me any questions about it. Even if they had, it wouldn't have mattered: I didn't really think I had a problem.

I always lived my life in a very simple way: Hungry, eat. Thirsty, drink. Tired, sleep. The pills fit naturally into that continuum of cause and effect: I was in pain, and I took something to alleviate that.

When I first filled the Vicodin prescription, I had a conversation with the pharmacist. "I gotta admit my ignorance here," I said. "I'm just double checking, but I take like three milligrams of lorazepam already each day." It was actually closer to six. "Is it okay to take together?"

"You're fine," she said. "These don't counteract each other."

I became accustomed to and then dependent on the cocktail of lorazepam and Vicodin, alternating both throughout the day. The Vicodin smoothed the whole world over; the two in combination were like a warm blanket under my skin, a soothing balm in my bloodstream. I felt indestructible. I thought, *This is the life. I could do this forever, change my brain chemistry permanently. Wipe the worry and pain clean forever.*

I went through a spiral of popping lorazepam and Vicodin in the morning like vitamins, maintaining that high throughout the day, then ending the day with more pills to relax enough to fall asleep. I was still working full time as a personal trainer and would train clients while high out of my mind. They were all losing weight and getting results, so no one complained. Just like my grandfather was a functioning alcoholic, I was a fully functioning addict. But I was such a pleasant person to be around that no one had issues with my behavior. I felt creative, inspired, motivated, but with a mix of bravado and fear. Fear that the bravado would be revealed as a mask, a chemically induced fraud. Because the outside was so pleasant, no one knew how rotten the inside was becoming. My giant secret was quietly swallowing me whole.

A rationale takes place as the drugs take over: You start taking medication to feel normal, to assuage some issue. Then you're taking so much that you're actually high; then you embrace the high and begin trying to reach it all the time. At some point, the high becomes normal. Not being high makes you uncomfortable, becomes its own kind of pain. It forces you to confront parts of yourself that you've been trying to escape, and it exposes your vulnerabilities. To someone who viewed the world as a time bomb—everything can go wrong, and then what will I do?—a pill that smoothed everything out was a powerful thing.

One night that winter, about 4 months into this period, I was at my apartment with Nicole and Rebe, a singer/songwriter friend of ours who lived across the street and was like a sister to me. Jayden was having a sleepover at my mother's and we had just finished a big dinner. I pulled out my hookah, which was frosted glass with a silver stem and cream-colored bowl. The three of us were non-watching a Justin Bieber documentary and leisurely smoking shisha, which is like a wet tobacco. I was in the process of one of my many attempts to quit cigarettes.

Before I even hit the hookah, a headache started growing in my skull. I'd taken a Vicodin and, 30 minutes later, the pain still hadn't eased. Rebe and Nicole were laughing about something and their voices started to get far away. My eyes began to hurt and I started rubbing at them incessantly.

"What's going on?" Nicole asked.

"I feel like a migraine's coming on, I think," I said. "I'm trying to catch it."

"You can't be hungry," Rebe said.

"Hell no, that was like a feast," I said. "I just . . . I don't know. It's like intense all of a sudden."

Nicole got up and moved to a chair. "Well stretch out and close your eyes," she said. "See if it goes away."

I closed my eyes and lay on the couch, their laughter floating upward.

Rebe tried to pass me the hookah. "You guys finish." I waved it away. "I'm good."

I hadn't ever doubled up on Vicodin before, but I figured maybe I'd grown accustomed to my dose, like with the lorazepam. I went into the kitchen and downed a second one with a full glass of water. But about 15 minutes in, I began to feel loopy and extremely fatigued.

I got up, wobbly. "Nicole," I said, "I'm going to go lay down in the bedroom. Keep an eye on me, I just took another painkiller. I don't feel 100 percent."

That is the last thing I remember.

I woke up with no sense of what time it was, or time at all, but there was muted light peeking through the blinds. As I came into consciousness, I felt a wave rumbling up from my stomach and I started throwing up in the bed. I darted to the bathroom, throwing up nonstop on the way. I was on my knees, holding the cool toilet for what felt like an eternity.

At some point I passed out. When I woke up again, I felt as though I'd been run over by a bus. My stomach was unsettled but I felt closer to normal, if normal included a wicked hangover. I slowly got up off the floor and laid down in the living room. Nicole got up soon after.

"What's going on, Quentin? What happened? There's throw-up all over the place."

"I don't feel too good. Lemme just rest it out."

Nicole told me my breathing had been faint when she checked on me, and that I had been out for about 11 hours, not moving, in the exact same position.

"No, uh-uh," she shook her head. "You need to call your doctor. Get an emergency appointment."

I didn't have the energy to fight her, and Dr. Barnes was only 10 minutes down the road. Nicole drove me, and when he asked what happened, I did my best with my memory while Nicole filled in the blanks.

"You're lucky to be here," he said. "This could've been bad. What did you take?"

"Lorazepam and a double dose of Vicodin."

"Two extra pills?"

"Yep, two pills."

He was baffled. "I didn't think your system was that sensitive to it, but ... "

"But what?" I asked.

"You had an overdose."

CHAPTER
12

WHITE NOISE

You can't drown yourself in drink. I've tried;
you float.

JOHN BARRYMORE

THE OVERDOSE SHOULD'VE BEEN A WAKEUP CALL, a signpost about how bad things had gotten and a mirror reflecting who I had become. It should have been that. But the mind of an addict is constantly constructing his reality—and his truth—in a way that only serves the addiction.

I took pride in my discipline and control, however counter that self-impression ran to my behavior. There was an embarrassment that came with the overdose, so over the next few days, it gnawed at me. The embarrassment hung heavy in a way that felt like shame, and along with it, dredged up fear: shame for my weakness, and fear of being judged and ridiculed. Riding back with Nicole from my doctor's office, I convinced myself that it was an accident. I'd had one too many Vicodin and my body reacted, so I'd just stop with the painkillers. I was thrown out to sea again, and—as was my habit—I just clung harder to the lorazepam.

But I found out pretty quickly that I had nothing to grab on to: The pills had lost their magic. My body had become accustomed to the painkiller combination, and it couldn't just readjust to the old ceiling. It took more and more lorazepam pills for them to work, and even when they did, I couldn't find that old sense of normalcy. My confidence was gone and the drop-off was pronounced. Adjusting to living inside the skin of my old self was rough. The fear came back with a vengeance, got stronger, and started to rise like a phoenix.

It wasn't just physiological fear—fear of attacks—that I had to keep at bay now. The fear was a ballooning force: the heaviness of my past, the misery of the present, the anxiety of my future. It was a fear of feeling itself. For a large part of my life, I protected myself from having to feel at all, so I didn't know how to cope with things so out in the open.

It turns out that this is a common fear among men, especially those who have been through traumatic experiences. It's also typical for those raised in a culture where we are trained to shut down our feelings. I was raised to strive for toughness, which over time and intensity, morphed into a kind of detachment. The biggest sin I could commit was to be vulnerable and show my true self to the world. I had to be a hard shell that didn't allow anyone in. I was afraid of my feelings, afraid of what they could do to me. So I always looked for ways to numb them. Throughout my childhood, I had to block out the pain caused by my father, the hole left there, the ripples that came from his failures and my expectations. When my relationship with Tamia failed and Chris was taken away, I drank. When anxiety hit, I took pills. Then I took more.

I was a grown man with two children, but inside I was still a 9-year-old hiding and peeking through my fingers, a 13-year-old building a shell against the world, a 20-year-old refusing to see people as people. When I returned to my lorazepam after the overdose, its effects were stunted. My body craved more and I went searching for something that could bring back that old self. And I found it.

A month or so after my overdose, my mother and I were invited to a surprise birthday party in downtown DC. It would be my first party situation in quite some time and the first since I'd started taking medication. I wanted to go but was apprehensive about all the variables: I knew there would be alcohol there and I wasn't sure how that would make me feel. Would the alcohol counteract my pills? Would it make my anxiety worse? I didn't want to shut myself off to the experience, so I knew I'd have some drinks. These were people I used to party with all the time at bars, clubs, each other's houses. They accepted me as one of their own and our bonding often revolved around drinking.

I wanted to open to the world and embrace normalcy, but in order to get there, I felt I had to endanger myself.

I was slightly jittery the whole day, so before we left my mom's house, I took three lorazepams.

"You gonna drive, Quentin?" she asked, grabbing her purse from the kitchen. I'd brought my car there but I thought we'd be taking hers.

"Oh, you want me to?"

"You know I hate driving on the highway."

I did. I'd forgotten. I was already taking more than my recommended dosage, but the pills hadn't really been working. When we got to the hotel and dropped the car with a valet, I reached inside my breast pocket and downed another four pills. Lorazepam pills are so tiny that I could just dry-swallow them.

The event was a birthday party for a former neighbor of ours, a close friend of the family. It was in a private room at the Willard InterContinental Hotel in downtown Washington, a majestic and historical place a few blocks from the White House—marble floors, gold trim, stone columns dropping down into the lobby like the legs of a god.

I took the outside-in approach, putting on the confident exterior in the hopes that it would drown out my fear. I was wearing beige dress pants, light brown dress shoes, and a white, blue, and beige dress shirt. I had on a dark brown and baby blue paisley tie knotted in a double Windsor, Kenneth Cole cufflinks, and a watch with a brown leather strap and gold bezel.

The guests sat in a theater room while we waited for the guest of honor. Then the party opened up with a dance floor, a DJ spinning, beer and wine behind a polished wooden bar. Some food stations were placed off to the side and I had a few chicken wings, but I mostly pounded red wine with my friends all night. Glass after glass after glass. At some point in the night, my memory cut out. My mom filled me in on the remainder.

She said I was alert but uncharacteristically quiet while we waited for the car to pull up out front. I guess I felt confident enough to drive and hopped in. As I navigated the downtown streets, a few minutes into the ride, she spoke up.

"You all right, honey?"

"Uh, no," I muttered. "No, actually."

"What's wrong?" she said, understandably alarmed.

"I can't see, Ma." I vaguely remember being behind the wheel and everything fading into black.

"Well, pull over, Quentin!" she yelled. I did and she took over. Somehow I stayed conscious enough to direct us home. When we got to her house, I was virtually unconscious and she had to drag me into the house.

The next morning, I woke up and drove home. Within hours, Nicole said I was talking gibberish, not making sense, sounding loopy. I couldn't remember my name or where I was. Apparently I was hallucinating, talking to people who weren't there, and unable to walk. Every time I got up, I fell, which freaked her out even more.

She called 911 and paramedics took me to the ER, where the doctors said my blood sugar was so dangerously low that had I not been brought in, it could've been fatal.

Incredibly, and indicative of how narrow-focused I was, the experience had the opposite effect it should have had. Not only did it not scare me, it reintroduced alcohol into my life. I chalked up the hospital experience to getting drunk on an empty stomach after almost a year of being sober. I told myself the most dangerous lie that addicts tell themselves: I am in control.

My drinking really started in the evening—mixing lorazepam and red wine to fend off impending anxiety. I was always afraid of the night. Whether it was because my anxiety was worse at night or the anxiety was worse because I thought that, I never figured out.

Initially I was downing a bottle of wine or a pint of Jack Daniels with some pills at home, just chasing that feeling. I'd get so intoxicated that even the fear of the night no longer became an issue, so I started going out. I embraced the party lifestyle again, staying out late and getting drunk with friends.

Unlike my pill addiction, which I was able to cover for and rationalize, I went out of my way to keep my drinking secret, leaving a wine opener in my car and never letting Nicole know how often I drove drunk and how wasted I was getting. I was well aware of the cultural stigma, had seen it in my own family, and I didn't want people on me about it: They just didn't understand, and I didn't want to explain it. Alcohol is not the kind of thing that's easy to discreetly imbibe. It's a hassle to be addicted to it.

Going out became the solution. Blend the alcohol and pills with noise and atmosphere, be around other drinkers, increase the number of hours in the day I could comfortably drink. I was working with some friends in the music industry on tracks and going to clubs to hear some of the new stuff that was going on, so I always used that as an excuse to Nicole. I was chasing this feeling that I couldn't get enough of, and on top of that, everyone seemed to love me. All of those years of being left out and now I was the life of the party. I ate it up. That gave me as much of a rush as anything. I went through a period of staying out to all hours of the night, hitting clubs where I'd hang with my DJ friends, and pouring bottles of vodka over my lorazepam in a constant search for that perfect feeling—what heroin addicts call chasing the dragon.

I knew all the DJs, the bouncers and security, the people in the VIP section—alcohol was regularly passed to me as a greeting.

"Hey, Q, come on over!" they'd yell from behind velvet ropes. "We got five bottles of Ciroc, help yourself."

I'd be pretty gone already, having taken a few lorazepams and downed a bottle of merlot before even leaving my house.

The alcohol would heighten the effects of each pill and would work as a stopgap when I was running out. Going through so many pills made them harder to refill and I kept running out earlier and earlier. I would go to my father's wife, who had been prescribed the same medication. If I ran out too soon, I'd ring her up. "Could I get a couple of pills from you until I can get to the doctor?" I'd ask.

"Sure thing, Quentin. Come on by."

"Thanks," I'd tell her when I showed up.

"Oh, I know all about running low. Makes it worse, right? Of course I'll help you out." She would put them in a zip-top bag for me and I'd pocket them and leave—hiding some in my car, in my home, in my bag. Making sure I never had to go without.

Lorazepam eased me to the point where my problems felt manageable. Alcohol was like a burst of white noise that wiped them out entirely.

I felt like the price for all this was nothing. I'd wake up with a slight hangover—nothing that some ibuprofen and a dose of lorazepam wouldn't fix. My body adjusted to waking up with that feeling. Some late nights or early mornings, I'd wake up in my car or passed out on the steps in the middle of the hallway in my building. I'd just get up, adjust myself, and go about my day. I'd head inside and first thing, go right for the lorazepam. Before I did anything, I would pop open a bottle of pills. That was breakfast.

||||||||||||||||||||||||||||||||||||||||||||||||||||||||||||||||||||||||||||||||||||||||||||||||||||||

One night my friend Reddz was hosting a party at a club and I'd just finished a bottle before pulling in. Security unclicked the ropes and I walked through. It was a club we regularly frequented, Corona and Heineken neon, a big wooden deck out front. The DJ booth was at the far end of the club on a small stage with a slick black leather sofa to the left of the station. Four roped-off VIP tables were to the right side of the DJ booth. There was no designated dance floor—people danced everywhere. Hip-hop, trap, and hard-core rap blasted through the space. Just deafening. The kind of sound that goes electric through your body. It was my element—an external space of noise to fit with what I had created inside of my body.

Sometime later that night, I was sitting in the DJ booth with Reddz while he was spinning. Slightly heavyset and light-skinned, Reddz had a tight haircut of reddish hair and waves, and a large abstract tattoo on his forearm. At some point, he turned around and caught my eye. "Uh-oh," he said theatrically, playfully almost, like, *here we go again.*

"What's that?" I asked. Lights were rotating across the floor and walls of the club, faces going in and out of shadow. The distinction between what was there and what I perceived was absent.

"You got that look in your eye," he said.

"What? You're tripping. I'm good, man."

"Uh-huh," he gestured at my full wine glass. "Maybe you need to chill a bit?"

"Trust me, I'm good," I said. "I'ma get some food at the bar."

I remember sitting at the bar eating buffalo wings and fries.

I remember downing another glass of red wine.

I remember moving on the dance floor, from girl to girl, having the time of my life.

I remember going back to the DJ booth and seeing my friend Ray, a tall and slim dude, dark-skinned with a low cut. Ray always wore sunglasses, even indoors. We hugged it out. "Hey, I didn't know you were here!" he said over the music.

"Of course!" I said. "Where else would I be?"

"I'ma get some beers, you want one?"

"Yeah, bring me one back."

I remember Ray returning with four Coronas. I remember this happening a few times. Some NFL players were holding court in a reserved section next to us, though I didn't recognize any of them. Ciroc vodka bottles on buckets of ice were placed like centerpieces across their table.

That's about when the recording cuts out for me.

Everything else after that was filled in for me after the fact. Many stories from this time I learned later, this one in particular. There were a lot of things that I just didn't remember. There are a lot of things I still don't remember.

At some point I headed back to the DJ booth where Reddz was spinning and Ray was hanging out. I was sitting on the arm of the sofa, eyes closed, zoning out to the music. Reddz watched me bob for a while, like I was floating in water. Then I slumped forward, my entire body collapsing and tipping toward the corner of one of the giant speakers. Ray noticed me caving, and he and Reddz caught me before I cracked my head wide open.

"Yo, Q, you good, man?" Ray asked. "You had too much? You need some water or something?"

"All good, I'm okay," I apparently mumbled. "I'm just going to go to the bathroom." I slowly got up and made my way through the crowd, stumbling and relying on the walls for balance.

"Watch him," Reddz said to Ray. "Make sure he's okay, don't let him leave."

At the time, I had a habit of doing that—hitting my ceiling and taking off without saying goodbye. "I'm just going to the bar real quick," I'd say. And then I'd be gone.

Ray grabbed some beers and then went to check on me in the bathroom, but I wasn't there. He walked around the entire club, which wasn't that big, and went back to the booth. "Yo Reddz, he ain't here."

"What do you mean? Where'd he go?"

A few hours later, around 3:30 in the morning, Reddz was driving up to his mother's place near my grandmother in Park Heights.

As he was circling around for a parking place on the street, he spotted my car. Pulling up alongside he saw me in there, head back on my headrest, passed out. The windows were cracked, the car was off, and the keys were in the ignition. He was blowing the horn over and over, but I wasn't budging. Reddz got out and banged on the window, but I was still a statue. Then he opened the door, patting me, then shaking me on my shoulder, and he still couldn't rouse me.

This was in Park Heights in Baltimore City, where I grew up, far from the suburbs where I was living at the time. Not the safest place to be passed out in your car with the keys in the ignition and the doors unlocked. I guess I knew I couldn't make it home.

My memory cuts back in here, though hazy and chopped up. I remember him dragging me into his mother's house: "Get up, you gotta walk, get up. You gotta walk." I was mumbling and grunting under my breath. In my mind, I was trying to walk but couldn't. My body would not function, as if the message from brain to limbs was blocked. Reddz dragged me up the brick steps, into the house, and plopped me down on the sofa.

About 3 hours later, I woke up. The harsh morning light cut into my eyes. I saw Reddz asleep across the living room, found my keys, and drove home.

I called him later that day. "Yo, what's up? How did I end up on your mom's couch? What happened?"

Reddz was quiet for a moment. Then he spoke, somberly, totally unlike him. "Yo man, we need to talk," he said.

"Okay . . . " I said.

"You have a problem. You have to get your life together."

"What do you mean? Where's this—"

"Listen to me. You have a problem. You know me."

I did. Reddz was a loose guy, a jokester who took nothing too seriously. This was the first time in all the years I had known him that he took concern about anything. He was never, ever patrician like that to other people. A live-and-let-live guy, through and through.

"You have children who are relying on you," he said. "You can't do this. I'm all about fun. But this is constant. I can't do this anymore. I can't constantly be watching you or worried about what you're going to do. You're not gonna make it."

My protests fizzled out pretty quickly and I just listened while he gave it to me straight. Until that moment, I'd only had my own perspective, which was warped and self-serving.

"Dude, I don't know what's going on in your life," he continued. "Whatever it is, you gotta find a way to get control of it. Coming to the club high out of your mind and drinking is not going to solve your problems. You have a reason to be here. Your kids are looking up to you. They need a father. Don't be the father that you had—be more than that. You need to figure it out and get it together."

I was shocked to hear Reddz talk like that. The disconnect between who I knew Reddz was and what he was saying tripped a wire in my head. It broke through my defenses.

And I had no argument. He was right—I was killing myself.

CHAPTER
13

THE PRICE

It is better to die on your feet
than to live on your knees.
EMILIANO ZAPATA

ALL THAT GARBAGE I TOLD MYSELF ABOUT there being no price
was just serious denial. Of course there was a price. And it was enormous. The pills kept me even and the alcohol kept me in a haze, so I just
never noticed. Lorazepam is a benzodiazepine, a downer, and downers
have long-term effects. When you're taking so many downers, you eventually become down, too. That heaviness would be there during periods
in the morning, buzzing in my ear, then it would creep in all day, like
something trying to catch me off guard. By nighttime I was swimming
in its waves and I'd just load myself up with alcohol and pills to keep
myself breathing.

I might have been an addict, but I'd always been a conscientious person. I knew Reddz, trusted him, and through him I was able to glimpse myself. I was willing to recognize I had a problem. So I tried to kick the pills, turning to the one person who had been there for me no matter what.

I walked Nicole through all the spots where I kept my pills—bedroom nightstand, wallet, car armrest, bathroom cabinet—and collected them into a single bottle.

"Let's try this," I told her. "I'm going to take out six pills and come to you throughout the day when I need one." I pulled out some cigarettes too and gave her the rest of the pack. "I'm gonna do the same thing with cigarettes."

"You sure about this?" Nicole was young, but not naive. She could feel that we were heading into uncharted waters.

"Absolutely," I said. "But when I'm done for the day, I'm done."

"I should keep them on me?"

"No, no. Hide them. Don't tell me where they are. Make sure I don't know where. The cigarettes too."

By the afternoon of that first day, my body went into a kind of shock. My body dragged and my stomach bubbled. I'd be up, then down, and the anxiety pushed its way to the forefront, like a jilted lover demanding attention. I had been consuming so many lorazepams a day that the low dose was unbearable. I had my sixth pill by lunchtime. An hour or so later, I was in a tailspin.

I went over to Nicole and tried to be casual about it. "Nicole, I'ma need a few more pills for the day."

She was at the computer and turned her full body to look at me, not saying a word.

"What?" I said.

"You told me this morning not to give you more than six."

"I know, I know. But I'm still figuring this out. I didn't realize how many I needed!"

"But you said, no matter what you said to—"

"Nicole!" My tone got aggressive. "Fuck all that! Just tell me where they are!"

"You're putting me in a real bad position, Quentin."

I couldn't even hear her. In that moment, the love of my life, this woman who'd always been there for me, turned into nothing more than an obstacle. Flustered, she got up and grabbed the pills, spilling a few into my hands.

The next day, it happened again: I overshot my ration and demanded the pills.

Nicole again protested. We were in the living room on the couch watching TV. She could see in my eyes that I wasn't going to make it to the next morning.

"C'mon Quentin, you told me—"

"Nicole! Just give me my fucking pills," I said. "I'm not playing!"

"I'm only doing what you asked me to do. Now you're mad?" Of course she was right, but addicts don't want rationalizations, we want results. Hearing Nicole point out what I knew only infuriated me more.

"Look, fuck all of that. Tell me where they are—"

"Quentin, you're not—"

"Nicole! Get the pills or I'll flip this house upside down!"

She ran into the kitchen and came back to the living room. "Here!" she rammed the bottle into my chest. "I'm not doing this shit again, Quentin. You're on your own." I had put her in an impossible spot. Once again, I was on my own, left to figure things out with no support. It felt like the only thing I was good at was pushing people away.

Forty-eight hours. I couldn't even make it 48 hours on a lower dose— an embarrassing truth for me to accept. The cravings were so powerful, so all consuming. It was like my body had turned into a giant, starving mouth. The whole experience made me so disgusted with myself that I began overloading again, just to push down the feelings of failure.

A few days later, I went to see Dr. Barnes because I was running low. When I got to the intake desk, the receptionist told me he wasn't there.

"What do you mean? These are his office hours. I've been coming in since—"

"He's on vacation, I think. He just left yesterday." A panic lit up my brain, but I tried to press it down.

"Well, when's he back?"

She gave me an exasperated glance and turned to her screen.

"Looks like the twenty-ninth," she said.

"The twenty-ninth, that's—"

"A week from Tuesday."

"But today's Wednesday!" I said, my voice rising. "You mean two weeks? I can't make it two days!"

"Sorry, we can't help you," she said. All of a sudden, I was a DMV customer. She turned her attention to the patient behind me. "Sorry, sir, if you could just let—"

"Wait, wait! What am I supposed to do?"

"You'll have to figure it out, go without," she said.

"Go without?!" The words wouldn't even process, I was so livid. "Hell no! You don't get it. If it were that easy, I wouldn't be here. I have a—"

"Sir, please calm down."

"Calm down? You're telling me I gotta go two weeks—"

"Mr. Vennie, if you don't calm down, we're going to have to call the police."

"I don't give a fuck! Call the police! Do what you need to do, but I'm not leaving here without talking to a doctor. I have panic attacks. That's what I come here for! This is the problem . . . "

Throwing a fit might've made me look unstable, but it was the only way to get through to them how serious this was. Eventually, she saw past my aggression and let me see another doctor in the office. He wrote me a 2-week prescription until I could get back in to see Dr. Barnes.

That prescription lasted about 5 days, so I had to go back to my father's wife for some more to hold me down.

The conversation with Reddz continued to loop in my head. The truth was so undeniable, a bright, shining light flashing in my face. It first made me disgusted enough to want to change. But once I felt like change was impossible, things got closed in and dark. I gave up trying to straighten out and just let myself skid.

I don't remember when I first decided I wanted to kill myself. It unfolded almost naturally: I got brazen with the drinking and the pills, taking more than I ever had before, hoping I'd go off the deep end. If I just kept numbing myself, maybe I wouldn't wake up the next day. Maybe I'd get behind the wheel, crash into something, and just be gone. Everyone would be happier if I wasn't around and my children would be better off without me. I didn't want to be a burden to them—it was the absolute last thing I wanted to be. The idea of being a weight on those I loved pressed painfully on me, lingered deep in the pit of my stomach, and nothing made it go away.

When you're addicted to something, you get by through imagining that you can quit whenever you want. It's why that first effort to quit is such a mountain—it's biology and psychology. Trying and failing kills the illusion that you can quit so easily, dispels the idea that you're even in control. I always saw myself as in control and only realized I wasn't when I let go and couldn't make it. I had to grab back on.

My depression sank me inward, keeping me in place. I stopped going to parties and seeing friends altogether. I barely left the house and just sat at home, wallowing and drinking. The few times I did leave the house, I'd tell Nicole I was going out but I'd just buy a bottle of Hennessy and sit in a car in a parking lot and drink myself to sleep. The partying can put a screen on the reality, but eventually there is no escaping. Like when you're crying at night. When you can't sleep. When you feel like your life has no meaning, no purpose. That's when the bottom rises up to meet you.

My depression had roots running back decades. When you grow up and feel like you have no value, like your life has no worth, like nothing you ever do is good enough, you get worn down by the criticism, tired of feeling like your life doesn't matter.

My mother had done the best she could, but she had a lot to juggle—jobs, duties, and identities, playing both mom and dad. My mother kept her eyes ahead, pushed me to solider through, and admonished me for wanting to express my emotions, following society's standards of what a man should and shouldn't be. It forced me to bottle up my emotions exactly at the time when I needed to feel them and learn their vocabulary.

So I suppressed how I felt: teachers telling me I wouldn't be much; being picked on in school; my father's addiction and imprisonment; going to school every day with kids who had normal home lives and two present parents.

Though a sensitive and intelligent person, Nicole didn't grow up with addiction in her family or environment; she didn't understand the power of bloodlines and was insulated from how bad things really were for me. She was wildly outmatched by what I forced her to deal with.

"Why do you have to drink all the time?" she'd wail at me. "Why can't you just take a break?! Why does it have to be all the time?"

The admonishing just drove me further in, a hammer whacking a stake deeper into the ground. I felt for her. She had left a cushy and relatively privileged life, everything she had ever been given and everything she had earned, and traded it all in for me. It was simply not fair. Knowing what I was putting her through, feeling it in my bones after every argument, just made me feel worse.

As a child, I had often thought that my life would've been better if I hadn't known my father at all, because I couldn't be disappointed by someone I never knew. When I realized I was replicating the same situation for my own children, setting them up for a life of disappointment, depression kicked in. By age 27, alcohol and pills filled in the space. My confidence and sense of self had taken root inside pill bottles. My feelings of validation were found at the bottom of wine glasses. I couldn't stop thinking that I was a failure. How everything that people had always said I would become—a deadbeat, a failure, a disappointment—I was. That logic became fatalistic: If this was the life I was doomed to live, if I was not strong enough to break the pattern, then what's the point of living?

I was 5'7" and could bench-press 285 pounds. I'd survived a shitty childhood situation, schools that wanted nothing to do with me, a life on the streets that would have taken other people down. How come I couldn't beat these little white pills? I tried to stand my ground, but quickly realized it was collapsing beneath my feet. Defeat loomed so large and menacing around me that I just didn't want to exist anymore. I was not who I'd always hoped I was. And I couldn't take it.

The cycle of thoughts became deafening and started blocking out everything else. I was exhausted—not just by the addiction and the looping routine of my days, but by my very existence. At some point late that summer, Nicole and I went to my father's house for a cookout in his backyard. It was a nice party, familial and comfortable. Even my mother was there. Pop had been out of the program for 10 years and was on the rise. He was energetic, talking to me about the new car he had bought and the new truck he was about to get. I could see everyone enjoying the day and each other, but I couldn't feel it. It was like it was happening in another language, one I couldn't grasp. I was tunneling down into myself too deep to absorb the outside world. My father and I had almost switched places—I was drinking a lot that day, after already having loaded up on some pills.

We were driving back from my father's house and Nicole was eyeing me like she was pissed.

"What's the problem?" I could feel it in the stale air of the car. Jayden sat quietly in the back.

She exhaled, getting the momentum to push it out. "I don't understand why every time we go to your father's house you have to drink so much."

"What?!" I said. "Why you always on me? I'm just trying to have a good time. I got enough going on in my life, I don't need you nagging me all the time."

"Nagging you? Who's the one—"

"I don't fucking need you to tell me—"

"It's pointless, Quentin! You don't see what I see."

"Good! I don't wanna see what . . . "

By the time we pulled up to our house we were both screaming. She ran into the house and called her mom, which she tended to do when she was upset with me.

I could hear her through the bedroom door, how tired she was of my drinking, tired of my surprise anger and my wildly swinging moods. She didn't get it—why I was doing what I was doing, why I am what I am.

As I heard her go on, I just lost it. I pushed the door open and snatched the phone from her, hung it up, and tossed it on the bed.

"What the fuck, Quentin?!"

"You don't need to share everything that's going on in our house. That's my fucking business, not your mother's."

"But you're not helping—"

"What the fuck she gonna do? How she gonna help? She don't know my life, only what you tell her."

"But you're not doing anything about it."

"What do you think I'm trying to do?! I'm trying to figure out what's going on with me. You're not helping!"

"I'm not helping?!" she stood up, eyes lit, more enraged than I'd ever seen her. "I'm the only one—"

"You're not. You're not helping! You're just—you're just making it worse!" I punched the door, made a hole, and the door came off its hinges.

"I can't handle this," she said. "I'm out. I deserve better. Jayden deserves better than this."

"Okay, fine. How about I just leave?"

"Good, and—"

"—and I won't fucking come back!" I yelled.

I went straight to the bedroom, to the little safe under my bed. I got on the floor and opened it up with my key: Inside was my handgun, a Ruger P90 9mm, which I'd bought years earlier for protection. I took it out, put a clip in, put the gun on safety, and tucked it in my waistband. I headed for the door.

"Where are you going?!" Nicole screamed at me.

I ignored her. She was underwater, her words not traveling.

As I got to the door, she grabbed my shirt from behind. "What are you doing? Quentin, stop! Where are you going?"

I stepped out and slammed the door behind me, hearing Nicole yell, "Don't do anything stupid!"

I got in my car and drove off with one intention, clear and focused: I was going to blow my brains out.

It sounds crazy, but I felt a sense of relief once I got to that point. Once I came to the decision, an ease flowed out of me, a peace emerged from the letting go. I had been feeling my emotions far too much, was oppressed and persecuted by them every hour of the day. Every ounce of pain and frustration I felt all of my life—the disappointments, the heartache of my son leaving, my father's broken promises, the things said to me by authority figures, the failures I'd accumulated—I felt it all so intensely. It all validated my decision.

I drove around for a bit, scouting locations, still slightly intoxicated from the drugs and alcohol I'd had at my father's earlier in the day. I was crying profusely, the world outside blurry and strange, when I reached an empty gas station parking lot. I went into the store and bought a pack of Djarum Blacks, clove cigarettes. I lit one and got into the car, put my head back, and took a deep breath.

I reached into my waistband. *This is what everyone wants*, I kept thinking. *They're finally going to see what their lives will be like without me.*

But the gun wasn't there. *What the fuck?*

I reached in the spots between the seat and door, under the seats, in the back, underneath Jayden's car seat—everywhere back there. I started to panic, thinking I'd dropped it inside the store somewhere. Just what I needed, a gun charge and some time in jail instead of ending all of this. "I can't believe this shit," I mumbled to myself, heading back inside.

"Forget something?" the clerk asked.

I certainly couldn't explain it to him. "Nah, I'm good." I peeked at the counter but it wasn't there.

I walked back around to my car, popped open the trunk, and stood there, mentally retracing my steps. It felt ridiculous.

Just like me, I thought ruefully. *I can't even kill myself right. The first time I actually have the balls to do it and I screw this up too.*

To this day, there is no doubt in my mind that if I'd had my pistol that night, I would be dead right now.

I drove back home and looked for the gun on the ground out front, but by then, my nerve was starting to buckle. I began to hear a tiny voice, getting louder,—maybe God, maybe me, maybe the universe in the way it knows how to speak: *There is a plan for you. This isn't it.*

I came quietly back in the house and saw the bedroom door, still off its hinges, perched against the door frame. The light was off, and I figured Nicole must be asleep. I went into the kitchen to get a glass of water, and there it was on the counter, shiny and black and louder than a bomb: my loaded gun.

Something—or someone—was trying to tell me something. And it was only in the silence that I could finally hear it.

PART III

TREE POSE

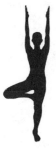

He will be like a tree firmly planted by streams of water,
Which yields its fruit in its season
And its leaf does not wither;
And in whatever he does, he prospers.

PSALM 1:3

TREE POSE IS A STANDING POSE where you balance your weight on one foot, while your other foot is pressed into the inner thigh of the standing leg. Used to challenge balance, it relaxes your mind and central nervous system. By rooting the foot of your standing leg into the ground, you are forced to accept the constant movement that exists in maintaining balance.

CHAPTER
14

MY DEALER

THE NIGHT OF THE GUN WAS A FLASHPOINT. It gave me the momentum and the desire to climb out—but it didn't show me what path to take. Knowing I needed to change was the first step, but it didn't actually get me very far. All I knew was that solving my problem was about control—accepting that I had lost it and taking the steps to get it back.

I had to stop wallowing. The fear, disappointment, ridicule, and shame: I had to face it all head-on.

It was a come-to-Jesus moment, a moment I'd heard people speak about, when God opens the floodgates and comes down to show you what your life is. That your life has value.

The first step was to tear this shit out at the root.

As I tried to do with everything, I approached it rationally. When I first had a problem with anxiety, I went to my doctor. The logical thing to do was to go back to him, so that next morning I called and made an emergency appointment. I got there, sat on the cushioned table with the thin paper, my heart beating a rampant gallop. I was going to come clean. Dr. Barnes came in wearing his white lab coat, his reading glasses on.

"What's going on?" he said casually. "Everything okay? You running out of pills?" It was the first thing he asked me.

"Nah, Dr. Barnes. Listen, I got a problem."

"What's going on? How's the medication?"

"The problem *is* the medication. I have a problem. I think I'm . . . I'm taking too much of it."

He stared at me over his glasses, inscrutable. "I don't see that being the issue."

My throat was dry and my voice cut out from the nervousness. I might have even stuttered. I was scared to say the words aloud, to give it presence in that room. I hadn't even admitted it to myself.

"I have a problem with these pills. I think . . . I think I'm addicted." The word was like a giant hammer cracking the earth. Just saying the word took a lot out of me—like telling someone you love them, which is the only other comparison I can give. It was one of the hardest things I ever had to do. Saying it to him was acknowledging it on a level that I had never done—admitting it to myself in a way that I had been avoiding.

It was a moment of humility, of letting go of my ego, of my pride, accepting that my life was not what I pictured it would be. But my doctor's response was astounding. He joked it off. "Addicted?" he said, the sputter of a laugh in his voice. "What do you mean, 'addicted'?"

"Yeah," I said. "Addicted, like I'm taking way too many pills." Rather than shutting me up, his response actually gave me some confidence to push forward. It made him less of an expert and more like someone beholden to things besides my best interest. "I can't stop. I wanna get off them. Find a way to manage without these pills."

He spoke like a disappointed coach. "Quentin, we've spoken about this. You're going to have to be on medication for the rest of your life if you want to be normal."

"But I'm not normal. That's what I'm saying. I'm addicted to—"

"I thought we had this thing handled. If you don't want a normal life and want to go back to panicking and living in fear—"

"But my life is in shambles. Things are upside down. I'm drinking profusely. I'm taking way too many pills. I don't want this life anymore." I was desperate, almost crying as I spoke. "I don't want this life anymore."

"Well, if these pills are such a problem, we'll put you on Xanax," he said. "It's not as strong as the lorazepam but we'll increase the milligrams. I'll give you the highest dosage that I can—"

"You're not understanding me, man. I don't want to be on pills at all."

"Tell me this, are you having anxiety attacks?"

"No."

"Have you been having any issues with panic?"

"No."

"Okay, obviously the medication is still working."

I was talking in a language he didn't understand. He made his living off of prescriptions—it was the foundation of his livelihood.

"I don't think you're addicted," he said confidently. "It's a natural progression that people develop a tolerance."

"It's not about tolerance. I just don't want to—"

"The Xanax could be the right solution then. We can—"

"No, I don't think you understand—"

"No, Quentin," he said firmly. "I don't think you understand. If you just stop taking pills, the consequences could be disastrous. Anxiety will be the least of your problems."

The words were like a knife to my chest. It was almost like he was threatening me, which was a confusing thing to hear from someone I had trusted so implicitly. I just wanted to get out of there and I knew the only way.

"Fuck it," I said. "If I gotta be on something, better the devil I know. Just fill me out another lorazepam refill."

"You're making the right choice. The responsible choice," he said, handing me the refill slip. I grabbed it and hopped off the table, anxious to leave. My doctor was a dead end. He gave me enough to hold me down, and I got out of there.

I'd expected him to at least recommend some kind of scaling back routine. But his resistance to the idea of getting off the pills, even when I came out and said I was an addict, was baffling. Well, first it was baffling. But then it was the opposite. It was all crystal clear to me. It struck me as I reached the parking lot that all this time, Dr. Barnes wasn't my doctor; he was my dealer. I recognized it, remembered fiends coming to me and saying, "Yo, this is trash." And my only thought was to keep them on. "I'll give you some of this instead," I said. "Tell me if it works better." In that office, I was my doctor's addict and he was not going to let me go. He was going to hook me for life because that's his job.

There's an old saying: "When you're a hammer, everything looks like a nail." Pills were his solution—it seemed like the profession's solution—and anything else was just noise.

I sat in my car in the parking lot for about 45 minutes and just cried. The one floor I could stand on—the trust I had in my doctor—had given way. My doctor didn't have my best interests at heart, and that threw me into a nosedive. I was cursing God at this point: Why was I saved? What do I do now? He showed me the night before that my life had purpose and here I was, back where I started—with no answers, no one to turn to.

I knew there had to be another answer, but I had nowhere else to go. I was too embarrassed to go to rehab, too terrified of what my family would think if they found out. I didn't want to be another addict on the family tree. I started to think this was all God's way of showing me who my father was but from the inside, seeing through his eyes, feeling with his heart. Maybe I was intentionally placed in a position where God was the only one I could trust.

In hindsight, I can now see how I turned a corner when I left Dr. Barnes's office. My fear of living life on the pills had finally overtaken my fear of living without them. I was a zombie, a slave to my medication, and I had to break free. What I wanted was deliverance.

When I arrived home that morning, I opened up the laptop and got googling. Dr. Barnes had said that if I quit the lorazepam, then "anxiety would be the least of your worries," so I got to work finding out what he meant. It was a small step, but at least I was taking control. I typed and read, typed and read: "generalized anxiety disorder," "lorazepam," "lorazepam side effects," "lorazepam withdrawal."

The side effects I came across didn't really frighten me. In fact, most were things I was already dealing with: anxiety, insomnia, nausea, cold sweats. What did shock me was the discovery that lorazepam is a short-term solution, recommended to be prescribed for only 6 weeks due to the likelihood of dependency and the need to increase doses in order for it to work; I'd been on the medication for about 2 years. I couldn't believe it. My anger and frustration kicked into high gear after that, likely clouding my judgment.

That afternoon I went on a medication strike, almost to spite my doctor. I rationalized that it was about will and desire and control. It felt like a purge, almost religious to me. I was not just going to prove my doctor wrong, I became engaged in a battle between opposing forces. I decided that I was going to emerge victorious, new, and clean.

But the body isn't like that. Not at all. I didn't know it, but I was like a train barreling full speed into a brick wall.

By dinnertime, I was getting crushed. Flulike symptoms had given way to what felt like a full-body virus. My stomach felt weak, and I flipped from shivering cold to burning up and back again. I laid around with no energy, a conflicted mix of restless and weak. My body had begun staging a full-scale rebellion.

On the sofa, laptop propped up, I scoured the Internet, looking for ways out of what was clearly becoming my prison. I was desperate—*anything but these fucking pills*, I thought, the heavy chain weighing me down. It was 10 p.m. My eyes were tightening and my head was pounding.

Nicole was lying in front of me on the other sofa, drifting off to sleep.

By this point, Nicole and I had been together for a little more than 4 years, living together for 3. She had threatened to leave me just once, and even then, I knew she was only saying it out of frustration. There was no doubt that my addiction was whittling away at our relationship, but she knew that leaving would've been something of a death sentence for me. Nicole understood that this aggressive, angry person wasn't me, and she held out hope that the me she fell in love with would return. But I was losing a battle that neither of us knew how to win. I was my father's child, a perpetual antagonist, locked in a loop and raging against the world.

I closed my laptop, put it on the floor, and tried to close my eyes. But my body rejected the stillness; I tossed and turned, flicking the covers off, putting them back on. When I stood up to get some water, my equilibrium was off. I couldn't catch my balance and I grabbed the sofa arm.

Nicole peeked over at me. "You okay?"

"Not really," I said.

"What's wrong?"

"I don't know." What could I say? I felt like my skin was falling off? My body was shutting down? "Could you get me some water, put some ice in it?"

Nicole went to the kitchen and came back with a glass of water. When she handed it to me, my hands were shaking so profusely that I could barely hold it. We both noticed the shaking and I started to panic, which made me panic more. It quickly went into overdrive, and suddenly I was inside of an all-out attack. My eyes began to water and my breath sputtered like the path to my lungs was blocked.

"Jesus, Quentin. Why don't you just take a pill?" Nicole demanded.

I ignored her and slowly stood up. She knew that the whole point was to not take one. Every sensation, every source of discomfort—I was fighting with my mind, trying to ignore what was happening. Just like I did as a child, I tried to get lost inside myself, trying to pretend the symptoms of the attack were simply not there.

"Quentin! Just take one pill!" She brought over the lorazepam bottle from the bathroom and shoved it in my face.

"No, fuck those pills." I grabbed them from her hand and threw them across the room, raging more at them than her. "I'm done with those fucking pills. I'll fucking die before I take another pill!"

My ego would not let go. I had been riding alongside death for so long, for most of my adult life, and I was suddenly no longer afraid. Part of me began to accept it as the only way to be free. I would rather have died on my own terms than in the grip of something else. And Nicole knew that. I left her with no choice. She saw that I was breaking down and dialed 911.

An ambulance came careening up to the apartment complex less than 10 minutes later.

"You can't do that," the ER doctor told me, almost shocked that I'd even tried. "You cannot do that. You nearly had a seizure. Did you look up the side effects of stopping like that? The withdrawal symptoms? Do you have any idea what could potentially happen?"

"No." Part of me was embarrassed, and part of me was enraged at being trapped. Hospitals and meds: the eternal sad routine that my life had become.

"Seizure, stroke, increased anxiety," she started to list. "Depression, suicidal thoughts, and death." Some of these sounded familiar, and some were new ones I could now look forward to.

"Wait," I said, trying to process. "You're telling me that by *not* taking this medicine, I could die."

"If you stop cold turkey, yes." Her eyes stayed locked on mine. "Your body is dependent on it. You can't just stop." I had been taking lorazepam for so long, so frequently, that 12 hours without it could have actually killed me.

"Go to your primary care physician and tell him to help you," she said. I didn't tell her that there was no way I was going back on that merry-go-round. I didn't bother explaining that I'd already done that, that he wasn't interested in helping, that the reason I went on strike was because of my appointment with him.

They released me back out into the world—a near miss, a reckless man who tried to break free of his meds. A close call.

Medical science could not help me, but I refused to give in. Lying in another bed in yet another hospital, surrounded again by the sick and the helpless and the damned, I just couldn't wrap my head around it. Why was I always landing here? The latest trip was because of my stubbornness, my pig-headed, fuck-the-world bravado. But I'd always gotten a jolt from proving people wrong. Dr. Barnes had unknowingly become another person lighting my fire.

CHAPTER 15

ROAD TO HEALING

It is easier to act yourself into a new way of thinking,
than it is to think yourself into a new way of acting.

MILLARD FULLER

I GOT HOME LATE THAT NIGHT AND CAUGHT a few hours of sleep. When I woke up the next morning, I had a newfound energy, fueled by indignation that gave way to purpose. Disturbed by the fact that this medication that was killing me was also supposedly keeping me alive, I opened my computer and got researching. I was a man on a mission.

People who have cured themselves
People who have gotten off medication naturally
Natural healing

Holistic wellness

Alternatives to medication

Alternative healing

I searched for hours, my eyes watering and my neck stiff, as I sorted through the collective knowledge of human sickness and wellness, the history of what others could offer me. I felt like a drowning man, kicking toward the shore.

One of my first finds was a documentary called *Fat, Sick, and Nearly Dead*—a title that snatched me out of my fuzzy haze. The bluntness appealed to me; I wasn't fat, but I was sick and nearly dead. The movie follows the filmmaker, an overweight Australian named Joe Cross, as his autoimmune disease disappears and his need for medication goes away—all in 60 days, and all thanks to a juice fast. Doctors in the documentary are baffled by Joe's transformation, as well as that of a diabetic trucker who Joe takes under his wing. Joe seemed like an ordinary guy—the epitome of an everyman—who through education and gall tore down medical assumptions and made himself healthy again. He willed himself whole again. The very idea that someone like him existed inspired me and made me feel that much less alone.

Later that day I came across a documentary called *Crazy Sexy Cancer*. Kris Carr's journey after a stage-IV cancer diagnosis had inspired millions, and I could see why. She battled against what was essentially a death sentence by turning to juicing, diet, yoga, and meditation. Her film focuses on the transformative and healing power of diet in curing diseases.

"When there are no answers, you have to find your own," she says in the film. Kris made healing seem possible, if you had the right approach and mind-set. "There is no escape," she says. "You have a full-time job. You are always at the office of healing." Kris reached through that screen and connected with me. She threw open the curtain on a community that I hadn't even known existed, one that was wide and welcoming to lost souls like myself.

Around midnight I shut the laptop and stood up, tight and dizzy. Rather than feeling drained, though, I was energized; it was like after staring at a wall for years, I saw an opening and a beam of light beckoning me forward. Invigorated, I hopped in my car and drove up the street to the 24-hour Super Walmart. In those blinding fluorescent lights late at night, everything was gauzy and a bit surreal. It was all so strange and distant, like I was watching myself. But the openness was liberating. In those aisles, a new mind-set was replacing the old and I could feel the changing of the guards.

I grabbed a General Electric power juicer for $69 and headed to the grocery section, where I snatched everything and anything I recognized from my research: $100 worth of celery, spinach, blueberries, cucumbers, ginger, bananas, and apples. As I rolled my cart to the checkout counter, the seeds of a new obsession were being planted. The checkout girl gave me a knowing look—had likely seen more than a few late-night rebirths—and I smiled back.

The next morning, I was up early and juicing.

Nicole came into the kitchen with visible surprise on her face. She saw me fiddling with this bulky machine sitting on our kitchen counter, the loud whir of the blade cutting through our house. "Quentin . . . Quentin!"

"What's up?"

"What the heck is this?"

"It's our new juicer!" I yelled over the sound of the rumbling motor. The enthusiasm of a young child oozed out of me. "We're gonna start juicing."

I had rinsed the vegetables and laid them all out on the counter. Nicole picked up the kale and froze a bit, just in her eyes. She was trying to connect what she was looking at with the man before her. I was not a model of health, but she knew I didn't buy random things on impulse. Something must have been up. I trusted she would hop aboard. We often need others to build momentum for change, and Nicole became my willing partner from day one.

I threw each fruit and vegetable into the juicer individually and poured each liquid into separate containers, mixing them in different proportions. My first few tries were disgusting, like spit-into-sink disgusting, but I wasn't deterred. I kept trying, again and again, and then again after that, mixing and matching with bravado until I tasted something I could imagine myself drinking every day.

I rolled through the process from terrible, to half-bad, to decent, until I landed on what became my go-to recipe:

5 kale leaves
2 handfuls of spinach
1 cucumber
1 chunk of ginger
3 celery stalks
2 Golden Delicious apples

As humans, we're creatures of habit and consistency. That morning became a hard pivot, repurposing the same impulses that had almost destroyed me. I channeled my focus and energy into something positive. Almost immediately, juicing became my new muse. My kitchen was my private laboratory and I was the master chemist. Early-morning juice replaced late-night alcohol binges. I'd pour my concoctions into my favorite wine glass and sip leisurely in front of my computer. Jayden was 3 at the time and even he got into it, as did Nicole. She pledged to go with me on any journey I undertook to get free and clean. Just having her there felt like solid ground beneath my feet.

Juicing gave me natural energy and clarity of thought. It also gave me an outlet to focus my attention on that was neither internal nor negative. It allowed me the freedom to be experimental and creative, and it was challenging enough to keep my mind engaged. I committed with laser focus to the healing power of diet and nutrition, educating myself about the food industry and learning what diet can do to both help and harm the human body. I was a sponge soaking up all this information and could feel the changes from the inside out—the mental leading to the physical. I went on a splurge watching all kinds of documentaries about the food industry: *Forks Over Knives*, *Food, Inc.*, and *Food Matters*.

I educated myself on diet's relationship to sickness and disease. I took a hard look at how malnourished I was, just by examining the foods I had been consuming—processed foods such as potato chips, turkey bacon, lunchmeat, ice cream, and bread. My diet was filled with artificial sugars, preservatives, and fillers, all of which have been proven to negatively affect brain health. I learned that red meat was possibly linked to certain forms of cancer and that cow's milk was never intended for human consumption. My diet went through a radical transformation.

I tried going straight vegan for about 4 weeks, but my body was also going through a detox of junk food at the time, so it was too much. I got hit with withdrawal symptoms: jittery hunger and shock from eliminating so much from my diet at once. I brought back healthier choices—organic chicken, turkey, and eggs—but permanently cut out red meat, pork, refined sugar, processed foods, milk, ice cream, and yogurt. The effects were quick and substantial: For one, I was no longer waking up every day feeling groggy and nauseated and sick, with a pounding and oppressive headache. I had more energy, not less.

Once the juicing and diet routines settled into place, I went after the elephant in the room—but wisely this time, respecting its size. I began my own tapering-off plan for the lorazepam, a gradual releasing of the beast, slowly prying its fingers off my neck.

Every day when I woke up—always a little anxious—I would push my body to the point where I could no longer handle the withdrawal. Like torturing myself. When I knew I couldn't bear much more, I'd take one pill. Then I'd stretch it, prolong the time between pills as much as possible, trying to distract myself as best I could. I'd take one, and 3 hours later, if it became unbearable, I'd take another. After a week or two, it became 4 hours and half a pill. This went on for months and months, a slow and deliberate climb to get my head above water. It was exhausting, one of the most difficult things I've ever had to do in my life. While I was fighting my addiction, I was also dealing with increased anxiety, depressive mood swings, hot flashes, and severe insomnia. I would often be awake for days at a time.

There is no such thing as a former addict. An addict is always an addict, for the rest of his life. No amount of green juice or alterations to my diet could remove that concrete fact. And I had never heard of anyone overcoming addiction without the help of a specialist or a 12-step program. I had my doubts; who was I to be the exception? Teachers and authority figures had drilled into me that I wasn't good enough, and I internalized their claims as my own. But the stakes were now colossal. Failure meant breaking a promise I'd made to my children—that I would be the father to them that I never had. It was a matter of life and death: I would rather die than live with the possibility of turning into the kind of father they'd rather not know.

For years I believed that if I acted strong, no one would see how weak I was. I'd be an aggressive man so no one could see the vulnerable one underneath. Too many men are taught that the only acceptable emotion is anger, and even that comes with contingencies. But I was done playing a role. I had been the author of a fiction that had constrained me and chained me down for far too long. The most important step in my journey was shifting my perception. The fact that the stakes were so high didn't frighten me; in fact, that's exactly what gave me courage.

After a few months of juicing, along with pruning out the processed foods and refined sugar in my diet, the physical discomforts of withdrawal started to dissipate. I was getting some regular sleep for the first time in more than 5 years, but my anxiety attacks hadn't really ebbed.

A central part of Kris Carr's healing in *Crazy Sexy Cancer* is yoga. That alone made the practice hard to write off. But I had an almost visceral aversion to it, based on nothing more than cursory impressions. I thought it was some kind of spiritual hocus-pocus or cult.

I frequently tell people that I didn't find yoga, yoga found me. It had never even been on my radar. I hadn't been raised around it, didn't know anyone who practiced it, and had no idea what yoga actually was. But then, when I needed it most, it seemed to pop up everywhere. Like the universe was trying to tell me something.

For instance, the gym I'd been a member of for several months started to offer a beginners' yoga class. When the class finally launched, I'd see barefoot people walking through the gym with colored mats rolled underneath their arms. They'd go into a dark activity room, behind a closed door that didn't bleed any sound. After an hour they'd come out sweaty, still barefoot, headed for the parking lot. I couldn't wrap my head around what they were doing in there.

At home, I'd see endless commercials where companies were using yoga classes as the backdrop surrounding whatever product or service they were offering. At Wegman's, doing my weekly juice shopping, I'd see tacked-up flyers on the bulletin board offering community yoga classes. I wasn't sure if it was a religion, an exercise, or something in between, but I was initially turned off by what it seemed to represent.

I did some cursory research, reading about its Hindu origins and connections, its praising of Ganesh. But I didn't hum and I didn't chant. I didn't understand Sanskrit, nor did I care to learn. I couldn't understand how standing in a few poses and praising an elephant statue with hoop earrings and beaded necklaces was going to help cure my anxiety. An Indian god that looked like Kool Moe Dee wasn't going to free me from my medication. There were too many religious components and connotations for my taste. I wasn't into the idea of praying to Ganesh and bowing in front of Buddha. I was raised Catholic, converted to African Methodist Episcopalian, and wasn't looking for another god. I didn't know what I needed, but I felt confident that this was not it.

On a Sunday morning a few months into my juicing, I was online, researching different green juice recipes while at my dining room table. The Internet is both a rabbit hole and a giant octopus, everything connecting to other things, feeding into other alleys—you disappear and get wrapped up in communities and worlds. I stumbled upon a YouTube video titled "All Hail the Kale Juice," hosted by a lean, gorgeous brunette named Tara Stiles who had her own YouTube channel. "My friend Kris Carr gave me this juicer," she said at the beginning, perking up my ears. By that point Kris Carr was my new muse, having smashed through my once-impenetrable walls.

Tara was a magnetic presence—and the juice recipe was delicious. In reading more about her, I learned that she was actually a yoga instructor, and I navigated to a group of her online lessons. She taught a specific kind of yoga called Strala.

She was nothing like the yoga teachers I had seen or read about. No Buddha, no chanting, no elephant, and no Sanskrit. It was all simple, straightforward instructions. "Down Dog," Tara would say.

Come on up to a high lunge

Low lunge

Side plank

Come into your plank

Let's do a pushup

She was direct and captivating, and I was drawn in. She had a casual, soothing voice and there was nothing foreign or falsely exotic in her approach. Tara made it all very accessible. She was simply the conduit through which I could tune in to my body. In simple phrases, she distilled the practice to its essence in a way that I could relate to and connect with.

For weeks, I'd set up with my little white MacBook on my living room floor and follow along to Tara's 7-minute lessons. After even a short time, the difference in how I felt was palpable. It was like the best shower I'd ever had—like a cleaning of my spirit—or a long night of sleep.

Tara created Strala yoga, which is about doing what feels good and not overextending yourself. It was the perfect bridge into the yoga world, giving me permission to fill up on only as much as I could handle. For the first time, I could let up and let go. In every other aspect of my life, my focus was on pushing harder, doing more, worrying about not doing enough, being told I'm not good enough, always pushing, pushing, pushing. This was about feeling, exploring my body and breath, my mind and what was behind it. It ran entirely counter to the previous 28 years of my life.

Instead of overly structured movements, Strala yoga is focused on fluidity and connecting your breath to your body and its movement. Its goal is the releasing of tension.

I felt an aversion to the rigidity of traditional yoga, the static posing that had to be perfect, that stiffness, trying to mimic the form of everyone else in class. Strala is about allowing your body to dictate and determine what yoga looks like and feels like specifically to your body. In that way, it embraced individuality. It was another way of saying *I am*.

Because my first panic attack had been at the gym, I had stopped working out entirely. Then for a few years, I was too high to bother going. Even when I was training clients, I wasn't working out. Yoga got me active again. To have that physicality back, that feeling of being in my body again, was like a rebirth. I cannot describe it any other way. It was that monumental.

I had been big into weight lifting for some time, but I barely ever stretched, and I never intentionally did anything to connect mind and body. After lifting at the gym, I might be tired and worn, often sore. Yoga was exhausting, too, but the residual feeling was the opposite: I felt energized and grounded and connected to myself when it was over.

I would practice every day, right after my morning green juice and right before my morning cigarette. Smoking tasted terrible afterward, like it finally revealed itself as smoke. While I wasn't sure whether I'd beat my addictions, I knew I was putting up a fight; whether I lost or won couldn't take away the fact that I was challenging it, bringing the fight to it, and not just waiting for it to consume me.

My goal in life had once been complete numbness. Yoga was part of a journey back the other way—not just toward feeling something but being committed to feeling it all: every muscle, stretch, breath, and movement, understanding the connections between my ends, my strengths, and my limitations.

When I told my mother about my newfound practice, she bought me a purple yoga mat from Five Below. After a few months at home, when I was ready to venture out to the local yoga studio in Midtown, I knew who to call.

"Hey, Ma," I said one day on the phone. "I want to go to an actual studio and do yoga. You down to try it with me?"

My mother has always been incredibly supportive of me, and even though she had never tried yoga before, she was open. "Set it up," she said. "Let's do it."

That Sunday we took a beginner yoga class at Charm City Yoga, a small brick building that reminded me of a small village firehouse. We entered this dimly lit front room of muted colors. We walked up the stairs to the beginners' studio and met Jill, our instructor. She was a small brunette who wore black yoga pants and a tank top, with mala beads around her neck. Jill exuded a natural tranquility, even in just welcoming everyone outside the door before class.

Jill had her yoga mat and Ganesh statue in the front of the small room, ambient chimes playing out of the studio speakers hooked into her phone. People tentatively made their way into the lime green room, picking up their foam blocks and straps and finding a spot on the birch veneer floor. Ma and I sat in the back and dialed in.

"It was pretty cool to see a mother and son doing this together," Jill said to us after class. "I don't see that frequently. You guys did great. I'd love to see you again next week." We both loved it and were there again the next Sunday.

Over time, I began to go regularly, becoming the early arrival sitting up front and developing a rapport with Jill. I was anxious to learn more, to explore the practice as far as it would take me. She was impressed with my focus and ease, and after about 4 months of regular practice, she suggested that I become a certified yoga instructor. It was the first time that a teacher had actually told me that I was good at something. The impact was enormous and it fed my desire to continue my exploration. It was a chance to take this further and see how far it could go. It wasn't enough that yoga was helping me; I wanted to bring this feeling to others. I wanted to master it.

I could've taken my 200 hours of teacher training anywhere, particularly at that studio near my Baltimore home. But I sensed that I should go elsewhere. It was a ripe time and home paralyzed me, enabled me, comforted me, and smothered me in its familiarity. Nicole was the one who first brought up the idea of going somewhere else.

"What about New York?" she said one day after dinner.

"What? Why?"

"For your yoga training. It's like the yoga mecca, it'd be a great place to meet people—"

"We can't afford that. It's like six weeks and—"

"Yes, we can. Trust me, Quentin, you need to get out of here for a while."

I thought about it while pretending it was a nonstarter. "I have no support network there, Nicole."

"I know you—you'll build one. Plus, Jayden and I could go with you and we could stay at my dad's in New Jersey."

I was looking for a reason not to do it.

I was still green in this new world, still dirty from my years spent in the pits of addiction. I still smelled of Djarum Black clove cigarettes and Woodbridge merlot. Still took the lorazepam, as well as muscle relaxers from a recent car accident and medication for my acne and some misdi-agnosed asthma.

I also still owed $30,000 for a loan on a degree I never finished, and I was still barely able to pay my monthly bills on time. In many internal ways, I was still a mess, still guilty about those years of selling hope to the hopeless, still guilty that I wasn't the father and partner I needed to be.

I was still trying to figure out where I was headed, what I needed in order to get there, and what would happen if I never arrived.

Fortunately, Nicole kept pushing, wouldn't let me be afraid or fall back on my old habits. It made a lot of sense, too much sense to not do it. New York was where I needed to be.

CHAPTER

16

my TRUTH

Between stimulus and response there is a space.
In that space is our power to choose our response.
In our response lies our growth and our freedom.

VIKTOR E. FRANKL

"GOOD MORNING, QUENTIN."

A beautiful, soft voice drifted in from behind me. I looked back to see Kristina, her curly brown hair wrapped in a loose bun.

"Hey there," I said. "Good morning."

Kristina, a graduate of the Juilliard School, worked at Physique 57, a ballet barre group fitness facility in New York City. She had become one of the few people in yoga class with whom I was building a rapport. Of the 30 students in the 200-hour teacher training program, I was the only man. As a natural introvert and a born observer, I tended to keep to myself. But Kristina, genuine in spirit and generous with her smile, stepped right over that boundary.

We were in a studio in Manhattan, gently tucked away in the fashion-able SoHo district, barely noticeable except for the Timberland store on the ground floor. I had dropped more than $4,000 on this program and was swallowing my pride by staying at Nicole's father's house across the Hudson River in New Jersey. Every morning, I commuted by train for training sessions in New York City, a place that I'd only ever been to as a drug dealer.

I was reintroducing myself to the world—or working toward it.

"How are you this morning?" Kristina asked.

"I'm here," I shrugged, a bit sheepish, mat tucked under my arm.

She smiled knowingly. Kristina grabbed her yoga mat from the floor of the storage area and made her way into the studio. I followed a few steps behind her.

I laid down my green-gray mat and neatly stacked my two cork blocks at its foot. I placed my folded blanket at the head and put a square block for head resting in the middle of my mat—the picture of organized and ready. Yesterday's 2-hour session had left my hamstrings sore. But it was a good sore. I unrolled my cotton strap to stretch it out.

Our instructor, Paula, walked in and sat down in front of us, a cup of Starbucks coffee at her side. She brought us all to attention by greeting us in easy pose. Six months ago, I would've called this Indian style. Now I knew it as Sukhasana.

I breathed in.

Time for class to begin.

It was still early in my journey, but yoga was helping me reposition my whole being in lockstep with something new. The teacher training amped up my commitment and focus, which emerged from a deep well inside me, one I didn't even know was there.

"I don't know what you all think this is, but it's yoga, not wrestling," Paula said to the class. "Why are you making so much noise?"

The room fell silent. Kristina, sitting off to my right, side-glanced at me. Paula's intensity had become a regular joke between us. I was being certified in a combination of Hatha, Ashtanga, and Iyengar yoga. Unlike Tara Stiles's Strala yoga, this was about pushing yourself to a certain limit, then extending that limit. Paula's approach was effective, but it was a struggle.

"Get into Utkatasana—chair pose. We're going to hold this for a while." We all grunted, a collective protest.

Chair pose is a vicious standing pose; your legs are together and your knees are bent slightly. Your shoulder blades are firm down your back and your arms are elevated above your head, externally rotated. To keep your pelvis aligned, your knees can't go farther than your toes. After a few minutes, your legs start trembling and your arms start caving into the force of gravity. Your weight is positioned more on your heels to keep the pressure off your knees, which also makes your thighs work harder. It's brutal.

"Ugh! I hate this pose!" a classmate blurted out.

"Does everyone feel this way?" Paula asked.

"Yes!" we all replied in unison.

"Good! You hate it because it's uncomfortable, right?"

"Yes!"

"Well, you don't get stronger by staying in your comfort zone, so this is the one we're working on. And this time, if I hear anything outside of your breath, we'll stay in it longer."

Paula did not fuck around. And we were training to be instructors, little Paulas scattered around studios all over the country. An army of Paulas.

"Inhale, arms up. Exhale, bend the knees. Draw your shoulder blades down your back," Paula commanded. "Press your tailbone toward the floor, keeping your lower back elongated. Shift your weight into your heels. Keep your gaze forward, lifting through your heart center. Focus on your breathing."

This yoga required a disciplined mind-set. We did as we were told, took our discomfort right up to the line of pain and then carved out comfortable space inside of that. We learned about recognizing what's uncomfortable and what's painful and truly understanding the difference. We learned that when you shift your attention from discomfort to your breath—your life force—you can endure so much more.

"If it burns, that just means your body is working for you," Paula told us. "Be grateful that it is, because it doesn't for everyone. Focus on your breathing, and remember, you get to lie down at the end."

In chair pose, I watched the clock behind her head. The minute hand was still, the seconds taking their sweet time.

I looked down at my feet and my legs were already trembling, my arms weakening and starting to lower. My shoulders burned and my heartbeat had pushed up into my throat.

Deep inhale.

Deep exhale.

Deep inhale, deep exhale.

I tried to keep my breathing consistent, a key part of yoga. It's the grounding you need to take things further. Your breath is the focal point no matter what your body is doing. It's literally the thing keeping you alive.

After 2 minutes, I was ready to give in and walk out.

Deep inhale. Deep exhale. Deep inhale, deep exhale.

Two minutes, 53 seconds. My heart rate lifted, and my chest felt tight. The room started to dip and then sway.

My left arm tingled a little bit, and my breathing felt shallow. Every inhale was shorter, every exhale came faster.

"Stay focused on your breath," Paula said calmly. "That's your life force. That's what's keeping you here."

Inside the faceless SoHo building, my arms were shaking, and my body heat felt like it was spiking. I knew exactly what was happening, and it couldn't have been worse timing. A full-blown panic attack, right there in the middle of yoga, in front of Kristina, Paula, everyone. I closed my eyes.

Three minutes and 46 seconds. My anxiety pills were in my bag. I was about to make a beeline straight for the door.

Just as I was about to straighten up, Paula walked over to me.

"Your reaction to the pain will not change the fact that it exists," she said quietly. She was right in my face, speaking directly to me, at me, into me. "But it will change the impact that it has in your life. Breathe!"

Deep inhale. Deep exhale.

Deep inhale, deep exhale.

"Don't let this defeat you. I want you to really feel this sensation. You have more control than you think."

She grabbed my arms and raised them to their proper position.

"Whatever you are feeling, take control of it. Tell it to back the fuck off."

"Back the fuck off," I said softly.

"I'm in control now," she said.

"I'm in control now," I repeated.

Under normal circumstances, I would've grabbed my pill bottle or called 911. But I found myself surprisingly calm, finding a space inside one of the worst panic attacks I'd ever experienced. And then the discomfort washed away.

But what she said stuck in my mind—it was the most astonishing thing I'd ever heard. I wanted her to repeat it, just to make sure I'd heard it right, but it already felt written on the inside of my brain. Rarely do we have those moments when words push through so deeply, so immediately.

Your reaction to the pain will not change the fact that it exists. But it will change the impact that it has in your life.

Paula leaned in toward my left ear. "You have to learn to find comfort in being uncomfortable. It's all about the sacrifice. You must sacrifice a temporary discomfort in order to find permanent pleasure. That is yoga."

Our eyes met and she winked at me. Then she tapped me on my shoulder and walked to the front of the room.

"Inhale to Tadasana," she instructed the class.

I just stood there, my body planted. I didn't move. We were done, but I stayed in chair pose a few seconds longer. My panic attack, the thing that had controlled me for so long, had simply vanished. Everything began to fit into place. My reaction had given it power. I had been a hostage to my responses, my own victim for all this time. The world doesn't tell me how to react, but I had assumed it did. Everything about me—my father, my childhood, my anxiety, my difficulties—all started to rearrange. This time, instead of running, I had allowed myself to feel the sensation, to go head-to-head with my disorder. And I was still standing.

Yoga wasn't interested in taking anything from me; it was devoted to bringing me something, planting something inside of me—my truth.

This was no longer about yoga. This was about my life.

In yoga, we struggle to bend and stretch into awkward poses, put our bodies into painful positions, only to find a comfortable resting place at the end of class. Lying still never feels so good as it does after yoga. It didn't take long for me to see the parallels. Only after facing the discomfort, feeling the discomfort of going past our limitations, can we have any semblance of peace. We overcome not by holding back or avoiding or seeking a way around. We have to go right through. That's where true comfort resides.

Yoga made me want to do better and be better. It was unlike anything I had ever engaged in before. It kept my anxiety in check and made me more aware of my strengths and limitations. I became convinced that yoga called me to do something; I just didn't know what it was. I still don't know. It's why I said to Kristina, "I'm here." That seemed to be the only fact that mattered.

Anxiety and addiction were never my enemies; they were my guide. They led me here. I control the truth and construct my reality. I know that now.

All these years, I thought my father didn't love me. In truth, he was like so many others, an imperfect person who lost control while looking for an escape. All of my focus and efforts to be different from him had led me to see him for who he was.

My truth needed to change. I had to realize that my inadequacies were a fiction all along, one that I'd help to write. The most important step in my journey was shifting my perception. That encounter in yoga class gave me the foundation for a new view and a new self.

The only things that have an impact are the things to which we give control. I wanted to become living proof of this, a walking monument to this fact.

Prove everyone was wrong about me.

Prove I am not my father. That I never was.

Prove I won't be chained to pills—to anything—for the rest of my life.

Find a place where I decide who I am.

What I am.

Find my truth.

Beautiful.

CHAPTER
17

WADING INTO THE DEEP

DURING MY TEACHER TRAINING TO BECOME A YOGA INSTRUCTOR, I felt my old self fall away. It was like a shedding of skin. The smoke had cleared, the cigarette aroma washed into the city skyline. I was beginning to see who I was, who I had been hiding from, who I'd been protecting.

New York itself was eye-opening, the ideal introduction to a new path and a new self. While there, I met celebrity yoga instructor Kristin McGee, who tried to sell me on the New York yoga community. She recognized me from *MindBodyGreen*, a lifestyle brand and Web site. I had written an article for them about ditching pain pills for green juice; Kris

Carr shared it and it went viral, and the new attention offered me new opportunities and relationships.

As my confidence in this new world grew, I tried to spread the philosophy and lessons from yoga outward into other aspects of my life. I returned to Baltimore after the training feeling light and purposeful, steadfast about hitting the ground running.

Unfortunately, the ground didn't come up to meet me. I set up a yoga program at my local gym in Baltimore. After a few weeks of classes, it became apparent that it wasn't a strong match. I didn't like how the place was being run and didn't feel like I had a support system underneath me, which is key for starting any new venture. No matter how committed I was, it was impossible to do it all alone.

As the weeks passed, I started to gain a bit more traction with the yoga class, but I still felt I was pushing uphill. One Saturday morning, I showed up to the gym before my paid class of 15 people arrived. When I walked into the group fitness room to set up, I saw punching bags and dummies spread all over. I went to the manager, Jason, to ask for some help in moving them, figuring they had been left over from a previous class. "Oh, sorry," he said casually. "We moved your class on the schedule."

"What! Why?"

"Dan called yesterday and said you couldn't make the Saturday class. So he took your slot and offered to shift the group to the boxing class."

"Wait, why did he—?" I was too livid to even figure out which question to ask first. "Why wouldn't anyone call me to verify?"

"Well, I couldn't think of a reason he'd lie."

"Unbelievable!" I smacked the desk. "This is incompetence, man."

"Sorry, but . . . "

"I've put up with enough and this is, it's just . . . "

"Quentin—"

"No, fuck it. Just take the class off the schedule permanently. I'm done!"

I walked out. I'd had enough. My writing had begun getting some attention, and I was being invited to wellness conferences, gatherings, and events in New York that I rarely attended because of my responsibilities to the yoga program. But if this was the way I was going to be treated, then I could no longer rationalize missing invites for an organization that didn't support what I was trying to do. It was hard to fulfill what felt like a mission when everyone else around me was just showing up at work.

Nicole saw my frustration and posed the idea of us moving to New Jersey. She felt like she'd have more support with school and I'd be able to explore the potential opportunities of New York. I objected, convinced that I couldn't leave Baltimore. But the longer I stayed, the more I realized I was limiting myself. Over time she wore me down, or, more accurately, I recognized she was right. When our lease was up, we packed our things and moved to New Jersey, making an agreement to stay with her father again for a few months until we figured it all out.

For the first 8 months, we lived at Nicole's father's house. Jayden had a room in the basement, and Nicole and I slept on a sofa down there, which was set up like a mini apartment. For a guy who had his own place at 19, this was initially a difficult thing—an exercise in humility. But it was a test, too. Was I willing to leave my pride back in Baltimore? Did I really want to start fresh? Was I willing to sacrifice for what I wanted?

Leaving Baltimore had been good for me psychologically, but it took others to show me that. About a month into my time in New Jersey, I was talking on the phone to my old friend Daryl, who I'd known since middle school. His was a voice I trusted, and he was someone who had always supported me. He'd actually given me a check for $300 to get my personal trainer license years back. "I believe in your vision," he had said. "I believe in your goal. I want to see you accomplish it."

When things in New York didn't explode for me as quickly as I imagined, I felt dejected and had been talking to him about it.

"Yo, I'm thinking of moving back to town, maybe to DC," I said. "Be closer to Baltimore. I'm not really feeling it up here." I'd only been in the area for about a month and there was something of a clash. New York was an aggressive environment and it triggered some of my old issues, gave me flashbacks of who I used to be—I was getting into arguments with people at the grocery store, or someone would bump me on the street and keep walking and I instinctively would want to throw down.

"I don't think this place is for me," I said. "Maybe if I move back—"

"Q, listen," Daryl said. "We known each other a long time, right?"

"No doubt."

I remember what he told me word for word, like it was this morning.

"Lemme ask you something—why is it that any time something might potentially go right for you, you find a reason to run away from it?"

It took a moment for me to process that. It sure sounded true, even though I was surprised someone had put the idea into words. "What do you mean?"

"You haven't even been there long enough to see this thing through and now you're already talking about leaving. For what? So you could end up back in Baltimore?"

"I feel you bruh, but, I feel alone out here. It's just—"

"I don't think leaving is a smart move. I think you should give it more time. Give yourself a chance, man. You don't need anyone to support you when God already does."

I trusted Daryl and his words had the ring of truth. My mother said the same thing a few days later. "As much as I would love for you to come back home," she told me, "I want you to really see what you're capable of up there. You've met quite a few people, you seem excited. Give yourself a year—see it through."

"All right, Ma."

"Remember, you left for a reason. I'm not going to close my door on you, but you need to keep pushing to see what this whole thing is about."

I even heard from my father. He called to see how I was doing, and I laid it all out for him: my fears, my doubts, my feeling that I couldn't get it going in New York.

"Don't make the same mistake that I made, son," he said. "I had a great opportunity to move to Atlanta many years ago and I passed it up."

"Why?" This was the first I'd heard of this.

"Afraid. I was just afraid. You have a chance to really do something with your life—don't be like me. You gotta take it for yourself."

They all lit that fire under me. I did think I had something to prove. I didn't want to feel like a failure once more, throwing in the towel and having to restart yet again. I was drawn to my comfort zone, but now I knew not to get lured into it; it was just a path back to old ways and discarded habits. I dug in.

<hr>

About a month or so later, I was invited to a *MindBodyGreen* event at their headquarters in Brooklyn. I was trying to talk myself out of going, saying I didn't need to go. But it was all a lie: This was the very reason I moved to New Jersey. It was all fear of the unexpected holding me back. The anxiety I had fought so hard to keep at bay still had an effect on me. So I put on a blue Ralph Lauren polo shirt, gray khakis, and blue sneakers and hopped on a train into the city.

The MBG headquarters was located in a newly renovated building in the Dumbo neighborhood of Brooklyn. I walked into a large, open space, a remodeled warehouse with concrete floors and tall windows. A colorful rug decorated the floor, with the three words *mind*, *body*, and *green* painted on the far left wall. The desks and computers were laid out toward the back of the room. Gluten-free snacks and cold-pressed juices were set up on a few tables. I can't be sure, but I believe I was the only black person in the room that night. The party was filled with the classic wellness crowd, looking as though they had been pulled out of a health magazine photo shoot. Pretty white women huddled in small groups, some sipping Prosecco out of crystal flutes, others drinking green juices.

When I walked in the room, I felt a wave of stares hit me. Making my way through the crowd, there were a few quick glances and then what sounded like whispers. I felt a bit uncomfortable from the beginning, so some of that was projection. But I was there, which was all that mattered. I was putting myself out into the universe, and even though it was not my typical kind of crowd, I had waded into the deep.

Later in the evening I was talking to the host, Courtney Gould, the founder of Smarty Pants Vitamins. She was asking me about my affiliation with *MindBodyGreen*, what kind of articles I wrote for them, what my story was and what led me to start writing in the first place. She was kind and inquisitive, so it felt comfortable to open up. In telling my story, I mentioned my experience with Tara Stiles's videos. Courtney interrupted and asked if I had ever met Tara. I said no, although I admitted that I had seen she was there at the party. Courtney took me by the hand and walked me over to Tara.

"Tara," she said, "you need to meet this guy and hear his story. Go ahead, Quentin, tell her what you told me."

Tara was wearing a short-sleeve turquoise cut-off sweater with blue jeans and was even more radiant in person. I had also never personally met anyone who'd had such a powerful impact on my life, but I pushed through the fear and told her my story. She immediately gave me a huge hug and pulled out her phone to take a picture with me.

After I thanked her, she shook her head and smiled.

"Thank you for sharing your story with me," she said. "You did the work, you changed your life. I just provided an outlet."

That was the first day I'd ever felt like I belonged. I felt at home, like I had found myself, right there in that room. That moment of reaching out reaffirmed my decision to leave my comfort zone.

Tara and I would soon connect on social media, and we began e-mailing each other. She invited me to come speak to her graduating yoga students, and she and another instructor, Rebekah "Bex" Borucki, took me under their wings and helped to establish me further in the community. Eight months later, I was on a flight to Los Angeles to shoot yoga videos for an app with Tara. We bonded over the 4-day shoot and became close friends.

Nicole, Jayden, and I moved out of Nicole's father's house soon after, into our own apartment in New Jersey.

I was doing personal training and wellness coaching along with some work and writing for *MindBodyGreen*, which had become my biggest family and champion. They invited me to be a keynote speaker at their Revitalize conference later that year, a terrifying but enormous opportunity. I accepted the invite, embracing the chance to share my story in a way that might transcend barriers, strip away stereotypes, and help others. The opportunity was frightening but also an awakening: How bad did I want this? I didn't even know what *this* was. I just knew that it was better than anything I had or was before.

Yoga taught me that it is not circumstances, but my reaction to the circumstances, that gives them power. Whatever I focus my attention on becomes my reality. It was a life-changing realization. It freed me in ways I had never conceived possible.

When I hold a warrior II pose and my arms are burning and I'm feeling fatigued, how I react is going to determine whether that pose defeats me or whether I find the strength to push forward. Of course the lesson reaches outward, which is why yoga has made such a profound difference in who I am today. Life itself is always evolving, always changing. We can either change with it and go with the current, or we can fight against it and become victims of our circumstances.

I used to focus on the fact that I was an addict and that I didn't want to be one anymore, instead of focusing on the fact that my addiction didn't determine or define who I was. I shifted my perception and changed where I focused my attention. I wasn't my addiction and I wasn't my anxiety. I started to live my life as a person who no longer feared his addiction or fear itself. I chose to become someone who had the power to alter his behavior and make that behavior work to his benefit.

|||||||||||||||||||||||||||||||||||||||||||||||||||||||||||||||||||||||||||||||||||||||||||||||||||||||||||||||||||||||||||||||

Yoga classes end in Shavasana, or corpse pose, which is just lying on your back, completely still. Some say it's the most difficult pose precisely because you're not supposed to move at all. It's all about the gap between what you did during the session and what you do afterwards, a moment of reflection and appreciation. After you put your body into all these difficult positions, you're able to find those 5 minutes of comfort in corpse pose. Once again, the lesson applies: The past leads to your reaction and your ability to embrace the present. And what we do in the present has the power to change the future.

During corpse pose, I started to notice this sense of euphoria. Over time, I wouldn't even know where I was, that I was lying down, that class was over. I was so out of it that people would have to come and nudge me, thinking I was asleep. "Out of it" is actually inaccurate—I was the opposite, so completely in tune with my body and my self that everything else washed away. My mind was settled and I didn't want to leave that space; I didn't know when or where I would find it again. I didn't realize that what I was doing was called meditation.

I began to study meditation and learned how to practice it. The purpose in meditation is not to have no thoughts—which is impossible—but to limit your thoughts. The goal is to go beyond your conscious mind, to find a place of enlightenment, to control the thoughts instead of having them control you. What we think becomes our reality; therefore, what we do begins with who we perceive ourselves to be. The goal is to free our minds from the control over our thoughts that we're conditioned to having. Scientists have proven that meditation affects the neurons and connections in your brain, and anyone who regularly practices it can attest that the effects are not just psychological.

I learned more about the breath, how it's connected to everything, understanding that it is our life force. As long as we have breath, we have life, and as long as we have life, we have possibility. When you can connect your breath to your movements, you're connecting your actions to your life. You're connecting yourself to yourself.

My work, my issues, my healing—it all came back to control; but I had to relearn what that word meant. You can't predict the future, but you can manipulate what it looks like by how you behave in the present moment. My tomorrow is based on the actions of today; my today is based on my actions from yesterday. Meditation taught me not to focus on the future, which is where I believe anxiety resides. Anxiety rests in the future, depression rests in the past, and possibility rests in the present. If you learn how to capitalize on and find comfort in even uncomfortable situations, you can maximize the present moment.

That's why it's called groundbreaking—you're breaking through solid assumptions. What you assumed was reality. The things that you once thought were the foundation of you and your world aren't even there. It was all in your mind.

EPILOGUE

OUTWARD

YOGA, MEDITATION, AND JUICING MAKE UP what I have coined
my "trinity of wellness." These three elements gave me the strength and
balance to manage my addiction, my anxiety, and then my life. Juicing
nourished my body, yoga kept me actively connected to my inner self,
and meditation taught me how to stay in tune with life's needs. I became
drug and tobacco free, and 15 months after the night I planned to put a
gun to my head, I reached one of the greatest days of my life: I took my
last pill.

I started writing about my problems with addiction and anxiety
while I was still going through them, and then I became a speaker on the
same issues. I bring firsthand experience to the table. I lived it. All of it.
I'm not that far removed from any of it—both literally and psychologically. Every single day I'm still faced with the idea of relapse, but the fear
of reliving that life helps keep me on my path. I remember very clearly
what the other side looked like, which makes me a valuable source. I can
relate on a level that others can't or have forgotten.

I don't view anything in my past as a hindrance anymore. It brought me here. Sharing it was the natural extension of that realization. It took a long time for me to know who I am and even longer to stand in front of others and confidently say, "This is me."

I'm vulnerable, but I can't shy away from it. For one, it's a reality. And second, I understand now that it's a source of strength. As Brené Brown writes in *Daring Greatly*, "Vulnerability sounds like truth and feels like courage."[*]

I focus on how far I've come. I am a guy from a single-parent home in Baltimore who was told that I'd never amount to much. I'm someone who fought addiction, battled anxiety, sold drugs, escaped death, and dropped out of college three separate times. But by the grace and guidance of God, I am here.

Three years after being diagnosed with an anxiety disorder, battling a life-threatening drug addiction, and surviving an accidental overdose, I am finally able to say that I'm not just alive, but thriving. I have been given the greatest gift: knowing what it feels like to really live.

My ability to overcome adversity reassures me that my life has meaning. I proved some people wrong and proved others right, reaffirming what my mother always told me: I can do anything. I credit faith and determination—along with the powers of yoga, meditation, and juicing—with saving my life.

I am determined to make my life count for something and feel a responsibility to share my story with anyone willing to listen. Not just for me, but for the countless others who lost their battles, or are still fighting: men and women who struggle daily with anxiety, depression, and addiction.

---

[*] Brené Brown, *Daring Greatly: How the Courage to Be Vulnerable Transforms the Way We Live, Love, Parent, and Lead* (New York: Gotham, 2012): 37.

I have gone from victim to victor. From addict to advocate. From anxiety sufferer to author, wellness expert, and motivational speaker. My transformation has not only inspired others, it has helped raise awareness for this debilitating mental health disorder and the overprescriptive nature of Western medicine. Years later, I'm drug free and spreading my message.

Mine is not really a story of escape; it is a story of finding freedom. But it's also about carrying my past—once a chain on my leg, it's now a torch I hold proudly in my hand, lighting my past, present, and future.

This is only the beginning.

APPENDIX A

JUICES TO TRY

WE ARE ALL CREATURES OF HABIT. I made a choice and committed to replacing my old behaviors with healthy ones. It's routine for me to start the day with a green juice or smoothie, and by increasing my daily intake of fruits and vegetables, I am able to provide my body with the necessary nutrients it needs to heal from the inside out.

Juicing works by extracting the micronutrients (vitamins and minerals) from fruits and vegetables, making it easier for your body to quickly absorb and utilize them. By removing the fiber, the body's digestive system doesn't have to work as hard to deliver nutrients to your cells.

ALL HAIL THE KALE JUICE

Thanks to Tara Stiles for this recipe. Add the ingredients to the juicer one at a time. You may need to cut your apple before adding it; it will depend on your juicer. Drink and enjoy.

    3 kale leaves

    1 large cucumber

    ½ inch chunk gingerroot

    1 apple (whatever is available or preferred)

ORANGE YOU DELICIOUS

I use this juice to help build my immune system and fight the common cold. Turmeric is a natural anti-inflammatory and a very strong antioxidant. Turmeric is also known to improve cognitive function, balance blood sugar, and improve kidney function. This juice is amazing either cold or steamed. Depending on your juicer, you may need to cut your apple before adding it.

    1 large orange, peeled

    1 piece (2 inches) turmeric root

    ½ lemon, peeled

    1 piece (½ inch) gingerroot

    1 Fuji apple (or whatever is available or preferred)

Add a pinch of freshly ground black pepper to the juice. Pepper helps the body absorb the turmeric.

GREEN COLADA

This juice is the first drink I make to introduce novice juicers to the juicing world—it's a healthy, sweet treat, full of iron, vitamin C, calcium, and vitamin K. I sometimes add about ½ cup of fresh coconut water to make it taste like a piña colada. The mint is a great addition. Your juicer will determine if the apple needs to be cut before it is added.

½ cup fresh pineapple chunks

2 kale leaves

2 handfuls baby spinach

1 Fuji apple (or whatever is available or preferred)

1 chunk (½ inch) gingerroot

4 mint sprigs

YOGA RESOURCES

EIGHT BASIC STYLES OF YOGA

Hatha: Hatha yoga is the most popular style of yoga because of its foundational roots. All other forms of asana (the physical practice of yoga) are based off of Hatha. It uses very basic poses to introduce students to the practice of yoga. The pace is generally slower than in other classes, and by staying in each pose for an extended period of time, Hatha serves as an introduction to the breath-to-movement connection found in all forms of yoga. If you are new to the practice, I recommend finding a beginners' Hatha class and starting your journey there.

Vinyasa: Vinyasa is a form of Hatha known for its constant movement and fluidity. Unlike traditional Hatha, each pose is carefully sequenced to go into the other in a steady pace. Vinyasa also connects your breath to your movement but in a more choreographed way.

Iyengar: Iyengar yoga was created by B. K. S. Iyengar. Iyengar emphasizes proper alignment, stability, and breath control (Pranayama). This style of yoga makes use of props (belts, blocks, bolsters, and blankets) to aid in each posture, minimizing the risk of injury.

Ashtanga: Ashtanga is a style of yoga that involves the synchronicity of the breath and poses to intensify the body's internal temperature to detoxify and purify the body. In other words, be prepared to sweat!

Bikram: Bikram yoga is a form of yoga founded by Bikram Choudhury. It contains a series of 26 poses done in succession with two breathing exercises, and is practiced in a room heated to 104 degrees. All classes are taught by certified Bikram instructors.

Hot yoga: Hot yoga has long been associated with Bikram, but it is actually any style of yoga that uses heat and humidity during practice.

Kundalini: Kundalini yoga incorporates movement, breath work, meditation, and chanting to increase consciousness and spirituality. This form of yoga is more spiritually based than other forms.

Restorative: Restorative yoga aligns the body and the mind through stillness, relaxation, and gentle movements. It uses props to help ease the physical pressures of holding poses so that the body can experience maximum benefit with very limited effort.

YOGA POSES FOR HEALING

Mountain pose: Mountain pose is a basic standing pose, which serves as the foundation for all standing poses. In addition to helping to improve posture and respiration, this pose helps to build confidence. Stand tall and affirm your ability to accomplish whatever you set your mind to while practicing this pose.

Chair pose: What I like most about this pose is that it can be done anywhere. Not only will your lower body get a good workout, but so will your shoulders and traps. This is the pose that taught me the importance of finding comfort in being uncomfortable. That's a lesson I will hold forever.

Tree pose: Tree pose was essential in easing my anxiety. By implementing a basic balancing pose, it allowed me to focus my attention away from my anxiety and place it on myself. This pose promotes concentration and awareness, and can be practiced anywhere—the elevator, in line at the grocery store, or while waiting for a train. Tree pose reminds me to be balanced and not so stuck in my ways.

Forward fold: Forward fold is one of my favorite poses for anxiety. It relieves tension in the neck, spine, and back, and is known to calm the brain to help reduce stress and anxiety. I tend to be very stiff when I get up, so I generally do this pose every morning to wake my body and mind. The forward fold also provides the same benefits as inversions, which improve blood circulation, help you maintain good posture, and relieve spinal pain.

Cobra: Cobra is a great pose to relieve stress. It helps to elevate your mood, while decreasing stiffness in the lower back. People (including myself) normally hold a lot of stress in their back, neck, and shoulders, and cobra is great for relieving discomfort in those areas. It also opens the chest and improves blood and oxygen circulation in the body.

Downward facing dog: Also known as down dog, this is one of the most famous poses in yoga. It is often used as a restful pose, but I use it to help with brain fog. This pose increases the bloodflow to the brain, aiding in cognitive function, combating anxiety, and improving mood.

Because it is an inversion, it also helps blood and lymph fluid flow in an opposite direction, taking pressure off the heart.

Warrior II: Warrior II is not only a very popular pose, it's also great for improving blood circulation and respiration. This pose also tones and strengthens the shoulders, legs, and ankles. And holding it for a while challenges you to overcome discomfort in a similar way to chair pose. In addition to stimulating the abdominal organs and helping to relieve back pain, it makes you feel very powerful while doing it.

Legs up the wall: This is my absolute favorite pose, next to corpse. This pose is commonly found in restorative classes and is great for relieving lower back discomfort and easing stress and anxiety. I also use it to help with insomnia, which occurs as a result of my anxiety worsening at night. When practicing this pose, I close my eyes and allow my mind to settle. It's a great pose to practice simple breathing exercises and meditation.

Crow pose: Crow pose is not only a great pose for physical and mental strength, it has served as one of my greatest teachers in patience and overcoming fear. This is not a pose that most people will be able to jump into. If not done properly, it can create the potential for injury, so there needs to be a level of patience and caution when attempting this pose. However, after practicing this pose regularly, I noticed that I started becoming a lot more patient in other areas of my life.

Pigeon pose: Pigeon pose is arguably the most popular hip opener in yoga. Both challenging and rewarding, pigeon pose is not only great at stretching the hip flexors and relieving sciatic discomfort, it also reigns supreme at melting away tension, both physically and mentally. It encourages us to let go, to embrace the discomforts of challenge and move beyond it. That's a lesson that I've applied to every aspect of my life.

Half moon pose: This is another one of my favorite poses to practice during moments of anxiety. As another balancing pose, half moon helps to improve coordination and balance, helping to guide my attention away from anxiety.

Dolphin pose: Dolphin pose is a modified version of shoulder stand. It has all the same benefits without going completely upside down. I started my inversion practice with dolphin, using it until I built the physical strength and confidence to try forearm stand.

Forearm stand: As my favorite inversion, forearm stand is a pose that I practice regularly to relieve anxiety and depression. It reverses the bloodflow in your body and brings your attention to your breath and your body's place in space, rather than the fear associated with anxiety or the despair of depression. By going upside down, you're literally changing your perspective and naturally evoking a sense of calmness and contentment. In addition, forearm stand also increases the bloodflow to your head and detoxifies the adrenals, which is also said to aid in decreasing anxiety.

Supported fish pose: Similar to legs up the wall, this pose assists in relieving tension while providing a great stretch to the neck, abdominal, and shoulder areas. This pose is also one of my go-to postures to connect back to my breathing during times of stress and anxiety. It encourages deep breathing and respiratory relief, both of which are important in minimizing the fight-or-flight response during an anxiety or panic attack. Personally I use a yoga block for additional support, which allows me to do less work and receive maximum relaxation.

Corpse pose: Known as yoga's most difficult pose, corpse pose is my absolute favorite. This is generally the last pose in yoga class and represents ultimate relaxation. After putting my body through numerous poses and postures, corpse pose challenges stillness, both mentally and physically. In my opinion it's the most vulnerable pose, commanding a sense of acceptance, peace, and relaxation. In this pose, you are literally taking a few moments to rest in peace.

ACKNOWLEDGMENTS

THERE ARE SO MANY PEOPLE WHO HAVE CONTRIBUTED TO this book coming into the world, and I can't begin to express how grateful I am. Without God, none of this would be possible. He has blessed me with more than I deserve and beyond what I could've imagined. To all of those who are reading this, I'd like to sincerely thank you for believing in me enough to pick up this book. Thank you for taking the time to get to know me and for allowing me to be a part of your lives. When I decided to write this book, I had no idea how much about myself I still had to learn. Through this process I was able to make amends with my past and heal many of my emotional wounds. I pray that you're able to do the same.

The intention of this book has always been to challenge what we believe to be possible. As a black man coming from Baltimore, I thought my possibilities were limited, but I've realized that the only person limiting me was me. I not only want to inspire, I aim to provoke change. Dr. Wayne Dyer once said, "If you change the way you look at things, the things you look at change." I live by that idea, and because of it, I am here today.

To my incredible agent, Kim Perel: Thank you for believing in me. You saw something in me that I didn't see in myself. Without your patience and persistence, I would've never been so open about my life. To my literary partner, Jon Sternfeld: I couldn't have asked for a better person to join me on this journey. Much love, brother! To my insanely talented editor, Leah Miller: You are an angel. Thank you for providing me with this amazing opportunity. To Gail Gonzales, Jennifer Levesque, Anna Cooperberg, Amy King, and the entire Rodale team: I couldn't be more thrilled to be a part of this family. I appreciate you all so very much! To Suzee Skwiot, Holly Smith, and everyone at Rodale Wellness: I am beyond grateful for the work we've done together. So much more to come!

Thank you to the entire *MindBodyGreen* staff. A very special thank you to Kerry Shaw. Without you, I'm sure that I would have never shared my struggles with mental health and addiction. To Myk Likhov, Caroline Burkle, Shauna Harrison, and Leslie Carr: I love you all. To my incredible PR, Kelly Taylor: You are an absolute blessing. Beyond business, I am honored to call you a friend. You are truly amazing!

To all of my friends, family, mentors, and inspirations: I'll do my best to name you all and pray that I don't forget anyone. To Wes Moore: Thank you for your work, your service, your encouragement, and your constant support. You are appreciated, brother! To Steve Harvey, Shawn Carter, and Oprah Winfrey: Thank you for inspiring me and showing us the way! To Gabby Bernstein and Kris Carr: I am beyond delighted to have you both in my life. To Tara Stiles, Kathryn Budig, and Rebekah Borucki: I love you all to the moon and back! To Brandon from Crunch gym in Garwood, New Jersey: Thank you for all of your support, brother. To Michelle Maros, Barb Schmidt, and the Peaceful Mind Peaceful Life Organization. To Kristin McGee, Rodney James, Dr. Jamal Harrison Bryant, and Crystal Steadman; R.I.P. Terrell "Smash" Taylor. To Swen and Sherida: I love you both dearly. To Mrs. Johnson from Sudbrook: Thank you for never giving up on me. To Tiara LaNiece, Ray Vic, Maria Mooney, Ray from Island City Tattoos, Eric from Sharper Images, Daz from Onyx in New Brunswick, the Sanchez family, Shellz, Mimi and Nikki, Corey Webster, Gary Whitehall, Arlene Wilson, Francilla Wilson, John Salley, Justin Johnson, Ryan Anderson, Andrew Aiken, Gelareh, Rebe, Chris and Matthew Featherstone, Tressa, Khiya, Tierra Byrd, Rachel DeAlto, Stephanie Abrams, Amy Freeze, my bro Steven Thomas, Gail Anderson, Kristi France, Monique Davis, Tyrone Melvin, Mike Hannah, Pixie Jackson, Martin Carrington, Teyneil and Ava Ray, Mike

Perrine, Danielle Diamond, Alvin Taylor, Anna Vocino, Thomas Huggins, Danielle Doby, Jason Williams, and Deanna Figiel. To Uncle Ronnie, Aunt Bet, Grant, Danielle, Chuck, Aunya, Lanine, Ronese, JaQuan, Jaylin, and Rasaan. R.I.P. Grandma Hilda and Grandpa Charles: I love you both beyond description. To Antoine, Lil Man, and Jamail Pritchett: I love you guys with everything in me. To my cousins Brandon, Rashid, Ruell, Julius, Amanda, Dave, Corey, Arnita, and Aunt Brenda. To my grandmother "Freaky Fran," R.I.P. Grandpa Sunny. To Nikki, DJ, and Travis. To Uncle Jay, thank you for stepping up when we were younger. Know that I love you! Roc, so glad you're home, bro! I love you, dude! To my Park Heights family, my big brother Reddz, Brittany E., Tenea, Brittney M., Big Mike, Topaz, Meechie, Lana, Cherese "Reese," Tarase, Jarrell, Kenny, Mike (from Homer), Erik, Big Josh, Dontae, Brittney, Melvin, and Fella. To Baltimore: I love you. To New Jersey: I thank you.

To my brother from another, Daryl: Dude, I don't know where to start. Just know that I love and admire you for the man, father, business-man, and husband you've become. I'm proud to call you my brother. To Eugene: We've been through hell and back, and I couldn't think of any-one I'd rather take this 30-year journey with. I love you, fam! To Ben: You believed in me when I didn't believe in myself. Thank you for all of your time, wisdom, encouragement, love, and support. I love you!

To my mother: You are the strongest person I know. Thank you for your unconditional love and support, and your unwillingness to give up. Who would've ever thought we'd get here? Your son has a book! How crazy is that?! It's all because of you! There aren't any words that can do justice to how much I love and adore you. Without you, I wouldn't be here. I owe you my life! You're my reason and I love you *so* much!

To my father: We've been through our ups and downs, but I'm happy we were able to let the past be the past. I'm glad to have you back in my life. I love you and never stopped! To Nicole: You are my everything. I wouldn't have made it this far had it not been for you. Thank you for pushing me and sticking it out with me. I know I'm a little crazy, but thank you for loving me in spite of it all. I love you more each day!

To Christian: You are my heart. Jayden: You are my soul. Everything I do is for the two of you. I'm blessed that God chose me to be your father. Know that I will never stop loving you. I push you so hard because I want you to be better than me. Know that it comes from love. You boys are my life! I hope that I'm making you proud!

To anyone that I forgot: Know that I love you dearly. And for anyone who has ever liked, shared, or commented on an article or social media post that I've written or shared, know that you are loved and appreciated way more than I can say. I wouldn't be where I am today had it not been for your love and support! Be well, and God bless you all.

ABOUT THE AUTHORS

QUENTIN VENNIE is a celebrated writer, speaker, and wellness expert. He has been featured on some of the world's largest health and wellness platforms, including *Huffington Post, MindBodyGreen, Positively Positive, Natural News*, and *Mantra Yoga + Health* magazine. He has appeared as a regular guest on *HuffPost Live*, discussing topics ranging from anxiety and depression to yoga and spirituality.

Quentin was selected as one of Baltimore's Top 30 under 30 Influencers, and he was recognized by the American Foundation for Suicide Prevention for his contribution in raising awareness for suicide prevention. Quentin aims to continue spreading awareness for anxiety sufferers, end the stigma associated with mental illness and addiction, and raise the standards of what it means to be healthy and how we approach healing nationwide.

Quentin's road to recovery has been publicly celebrated by notable figures in the world of wellness and beyond. His transformation has inspired thousands worldwide and has raised global awareness of anxiety, depression, and addiction. He is living proof that during our weakest moments, we have the power and ability to unlock unimaginable strength.

JON STERNFELD is a writer and editor who lives in New York. He cowrote *Crisis Point: Why We Must—And How We Can—Overcome Our Broken Politics in Washington and Across America* with Senators Tom Daschle and Trent Lott, *A Stone of Hope: A Memoir* with Jim St. Germain, and *Steer: Using the Surprising Power of Anxiety in Life, Love, and Work* with Alicia H. Clark.

INDEX

Boldface references indicate photographs.